Serious Illness in the Classroom

Serious Illness in the Classroom
An Educator's Resource

Andrea L. Mesec

Medical Advisor
Charles H. Fraser, M.D.

1997
Teacher Ideas Press
A Division of
Libraries Unlimited, Inc.
Englewood, Colorado

TEACHER IDEAS PRESS
A Division of
Libraries Unlimited, Inc.
P.O. Box 6633
Englewood, CO 80155-6633
1-800-237-6124

Production Editor: Kevin W. Perizzolo
Copy Editor: Louise C. Tonneson
Proofreader: Ryan Goldberg
Typesetter: Michael Florman

Library of Congress Cataloging-in-Publication Data

Mesec, Andrea L., 1969-
    Serious illness in the classroom : an educator's resource / Andrea
L. Mesec.
    xv, 117 p. 17x25 cm.
    Includes bibliographical references (p. 115) and index.
    ISBN 1-56308-416-3
    1. School children--Health and hygiene--United States--Handbooks,
manuals, etc. 2. Diseases--United States--Handbooks, manuals, etc.
3. Classroom management--United States--Handbooks, manuals etc.
4. Sick children--United States--Psychology--Handbooks, manuals.
5. School health services--United States--Handbooks, manuals, etc.
I. Fraser, Charles H., 1928-   . II. Title.
LB3409.U5M47 1997
371.7'12--dc20   96-41965
                                                              CIP

To my Family and Danny

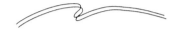

Contents

x Contents

Preface

Serious Illness in the Classroom is the result of an experience during my first year as a full time teacher. One of my students that year was diagnosed with a potentially life-threatening illness. I was overwhelmed. The idea that I was to be the responsible adult in this child's life for six hours every day was unnerving. Concern compelled me to search for information that would explain how to assist this child. My greatest challenge actually led me to locate information that was applicable to the classroom.

My intent in writing this book is to put all of that hard earned information—a hodgepodge of pamphlets, books, articles, and notes—in one convenient location. I hope it will ease some of the stress other classroom teachers might feel when they are teaching a child with a serious illness. This guidebook is not intended to be a text full of the latest medical breakthroughs (although I have attempted to make it as current as possible). Rather, it is meant to provide basic information about these illnesses, including facts that will help to create a safer environment for the child at school, and ideas on how to share this information with a class.

Serious Illness in the Classroom should be considered a tool for educators that will assist them as they work with students who are suffering from a serious illness, and for others who support them, such as parents, other teachers, school personnel, and classmates. It is a source that can minimize the negative impact on those students' education.

I hope that the lesson ideas included in this book will help teachers to share the facts about these illnesses. I believe this will lead to more thoughtful attitudes, and an understanding of the needs of a student with a serious illness.

Every effort has been made to ensure that the medical information presented in this book is accurate. The author and publisher, however, cannot accept responsibility for, or consequences resulting from, the application of the information in this book, and make no warranty, express or implied. If any of your students are under the care of a doctor and receive advice contrary to that offered in this book, follow the doctor's advice. The characteristics of the student's problem can then be taken into account. Always follow the school nurse's instructions as well.

Acknowledgments

I would like to acknowledge Suzanne Barchers for her encouragement in pursuing this project, Sarah and Kathy for their partnership in the initial assignment that led to a chapter of this book, Corel Software for their wonderful clip art, everyone at Teacher Ideas Press for all their help, Dr. Mijer for his guidance, Dr. Charles H. Fraser for his time and knowledge, and finally, my family for their support.

Introduction

The onset of a serious illness affects the whole child. The teacher will become aware that illness can, and often does, affect a student in more ways than physical health. Physically, the student will have much to deal with and understand. He/she must learn to monitor their body and respond appropriately to its needs, as well as self-regulate a daily medical health plan as much as possible.

Change is stressful. The change from a healthy child to one with an illness can lead to emotional upset and consequently, behavior problems. It becomes important to help the child maintain a positive self image. By encouraging the entire class to understand the illness from a scientific standpoint, the children should find continued acceptance within their peer group. Such acceptance should contribute to continued healthy social development. Additionally, the scientific perspective will help to negate possible interpretation of the illness as some kind of punishment.

Changes that occur in a student's life, such as an illness, can affect them academically. Teachers will react differently to the news of the illness, and such reactions affect the child. A teacher's expectations are often fulfilled in their students. Therefore, if teachers lower their expectations because of an illness, the student might just prove them correct. Luckily, most children are resilient. Nevertheless, a teacher's responsibility is to assist in the educational growth of all students. Educators must do all that is possible to keep the illness from negatively affecting the development of the child. It is generally most helpful to the child if expectations, both behavioral and academic, are maintained at a challenging level.

If illness or hospitalization causes a child to miss school, the child may be very apprehensive about returning to class. Being worried about unfinished assignments, tests, peers, teachers, or other problems is not uncommon. The best approach for the child who has missed an extended period of time away from school is encouragement to return as soon as possible. Adaptations should be made to the schedule or workload to facilitate the child's return.

It is important, when the child returns to school, to provide him with the safest environment possible. The faculty and staff at the school should be adequately informed in case of an emergency. All necessary information about the child should be organized and placed in the classroom, school clinic, office, and in a substitute teacher folder. It is also a good idea to have an extra copy in a field trip folder. There are support materials located at the back of this book to help gather the necessary information and permissions from the student's family.

Chapter 1
Allergies

An Allergy is an extreme sensitivity of the immune system to something that is normally harmless. The various Allergies are often named after the substance, the Allergen, that causes the allergic reaction. Allergies are noncontagious conditions that are different for each individual. These differences are created because each immune system learns each Allergy individually.

DESCRIPTION

Allergies are the result of an unnecessary immune system reaction. The purpose of the immune system is to attack and destroy infections and foreign substances in the body. The system produces chemicals called Antibodies that identify specific dangers and alert the body's defenses. When the system mistakenly identifies a harmless substance as something dangerous and attacks it, that substance is called an Allergen and the unnecessary reaction, an Allergy.

It takes two different exposures to an Allergen for an allergic reaction to take place. During the first exposure, the immune system mis-educates itself as to the harm of the substance. Antibodies to the Allergen are then produced and stored. While in storage, they have no effect. When the second exposure to an Allergen occurs, these Antibodies are released. These chemicals fiercely attack the Allergen, causing an allergic reaction. This will occur at each subsequent exposure.

An Allergy can affect any system in the body. Some commonly affected areas are the respiratory system, the digestive system, blood vessels, and the skin. Allergic reactions can occur away from, or at the site of contact.

Allergic reactions vary greatly in their severity. The most serious type of reaction is called Anaphylaxis, or Anaphylactic Shock. This reaction involves the entire body and is considered a medical emergency.

Anaphylactic Shock victims exhibit anxiety, itching, flushing, headache, nausea, vomiting, sneezing, coughing, abdominal cramps, hives, swelling (especially of the Respiratory passages and blood vessels), diarrhea, shortness of breath, wheezing, larynx spasms, low blood pressure, convulsions, or loss of consciousness. Anaphylaxis can result in death. Allergens that are commonly associated with Anaphylaxis are insect venoms, penicillin, fish, peanuts, eggs, and seeds.

The fundamental cause of Allergies is unknown, but the tendency for it does run in families. There are three main types of Allergies, each named after the kinds of Allergens that cause them.

Hay Fever

Hay fever is the most common Allergy. It is an inflammation of the mucus membranes in the nose, which is caused by Allergens in the air we breath. If the Allergen is seasonal, such as pollen from trees, grasses, weeds, or mold spores, it is called seasonal allergic rhinitis. If the Allergen is present throughout the year, like house dust, animal danders, or odors, it is called perennial allergic rhinitis.

Food Allergies

Food Allergies are reactions by the immune system to the ingestion of a particular food or food additive.

Hives

Hives are flat and irregularly shaped, intensely itchy swellings of the skin or mucus membranes that usually occur in groups. They vary in size from a fourth of an inch to one foot in diameter, last one to six hours, and then fade, usually leaving no trace. As they are forming, hives itch, burn, and/or sting.

SYMPTOMS

There are many different symptoms that accompany an allergic reaction. Often they go undiagnosed as Allergies because they are assumed to be caused by something else. Some of the symptoms of Allergies appear below.

General Symptoms

- headaches
- runny eyes, nose

- difficulty breathing
- nausea
- diarrhea
- skin rash
- stomachache

Skin Allergy Symptoms

- rash or scaly skin (Eczema)
- blistery, itchy, inflamed skin (contact dermatitis)
- red, swollen, irritated skin (hives, urticaria)

Eye and Ear Allergy Symptoms

- red, swollen eyes, nose, or eyelids
- runny eyes and nose
- soreness
- fluid in the ear
- difficulty hearing
- stuffiness
- sneezing

Food Allergy Symptoms

- stomachache
- nausea
- vomiting
- diarrhea
- swelling in and around mouth
- skin rash
- wheezing

Other Possible Symptoms

- depression
- anxiety
- headaches
- hyperactivity
- convulsions
- migraines
- Anaphylaxis

DIAGNOSIS

 Diagnosing Allergies can be very difficult, especially if the allergic reaction is delayed. There are some clues that can make diagnosis easier, including a seasonal or predictable appearance of symptoms. Other clues are discovered through the use of diaries, in which the person's symptoms are recorded. In this way, the Allergy can be diagnosed through the process of elimination. This is usually the case in diagnosing food Allergies. The patient is put on a strict diet. As different foods are added to the diet, the doctor and patient watch for symptoms. If they occur, an Allergy is determined to be present. There are also some tests that can be performed to determine what the Allergy may be.

Skin Test

This is used primarily to test for airborne and skin Allergies. It involves up to forty skin pricks done by a needle, often on the patient's back. A solution containing a suspected Allergen is then dropped onto the pricked spot. If a round red welt, or wheal, appears on the pricked spot within approximately fifteen minutes, it is considered to be a positive result, and the patient is diagnosed as allergic to that particular substance.

Double Blind Food Allergy Test

This test uses capsules that contain either the suspected food Allergen or a placebo—a substance that is known to be harmless. The capsules are ingested at different times and symptoms are monitored. Neither the doctor nor the patient are aware of which capsule contains the Allergen. If there is a reaction, a diagnosis is made.

Radioimmunosorbant Assay Test (RAST)

This test analyzes a sample of the patient's blood for Antibodies to certain substances. If Antibodies to an Allergen are present, then a diagnosis can be made.

TREATMENT

There are a variety of treatments available for Allergy patients. The treatments fall into three categories: avoidance, immunotherapy, and medications.

Avoidance

The patient attempts to avoid all contact with the Allergen(s). This is the only treatment for food Allergies.

Immunotherapy (Allergy shots)

This involves a series of injections that contain a small amount of an Allergen. The shots are administered once or twice a week in increasing doses, until reaching the highest dose that is possible without bringing on a serious allergic reaction. This level is called the maintenance level. Shots are usually continued at the maintenance level every two to four weeks.

Medication

Prescribed.
These vary from strong doses of over-the-counter medications to steroids.
Over the counter.
These include antihistamines and decongestants.
Injections.
This is an emergency treatment for Anaphylaxis. If necessary, it is carried at all times. (For example: a bee sting is unpredictable and could happen at anytime.)

WARNING SIGNS

All of the symptoms listed so far are warning signs that a person is suffering from an allergic reaction. There are some symptoms that signify a possible emergency. These are the symptoms of Anaphylaxis. If a person is considered to be at high risk for Anaphylactic Shock, they will carry a single shot dose of a steroid for the emergency treatment of the symptoms. The shot should be administered at the appearance of severe symptoms. Emergency personnel should also be called.

- severe itching all over
- severe rash
- swelling (especially of the eyes, tongue, and throat)
- loss of consciousness

COMMON ALLERGENS

- pollens
- mold spores
- house dust
- dust mites
- animal danders
- foods–nuts, shellfish, dairy products
- insect bites
- metals

CLASSROOM LESSON IDEAS

Lesson 1

What Are Allergies?

Educational Objective:

To introduce students to the term Allergy and its definition.

Materials:

Butcher paper set up as below.

K	W	L
What I Know	**What I Want to Know**	**What I Learned**

Procedure:

1. Begin the lesson by asking the class to brainstorm on what they already know about Allergies.

2. Fill out the "What I Know" section of the KWL chart with their suggestions.

3. Ask the students what their questions are concerning Allergies.

4. List these questions in the "What I Want to Know" section of the chart.

The next part of the lesson depends on the age of the students. Younger students can have their questions answered by the teacher, a visiting medical professional, or through a book read aloud to them. Older students may be given materials from which they can find the answers to their questions on their own. (This chapter on Allergies should be helpful.)

This activity can be conducted in cooperative learning groups or individually. After the students fill out their own "What I Learned" sections, the groups can reconvene and discuss their questions and answers. This ensures that the students draw correct conclusions about Allergies.

Closure

Discuss with the students why it might be important for them to know about Allergies, and how they can be supportive of a classmate with an Allergy.

Lesson 2

An Allergic Reaction—
Reacting to an Emergency

Educational objectives:

1. To compare an allergic reaction to a planned response to an emergency.
2. To develop the concept of how allergic reactions are unnecessary reactions.
3. To review an emergency response used in the school.

Expectations:

1. Students work in their groups.
2. Students speak at a whisper.
3. Students remain at their own tables.

Materials:

1. The school's fire drill procedure.
2. The blank emergency plan outline found at the end of this lesson. (page 10)
3. The example fire drill map found at the end of this lesson. (page 11)

Exploration Phase

First, remind students that the fire drill procedure is a planned response to an emergency. Then give each group of students a blank outline of an emergency plan. On it, ask the students to draw a response to an emergency situation.

The students can be given a specific procedure to outline, such as evacuating all students from the classrooms, while still keeping them within the building. Another option is to give the students a scenario from which they create the planned reaction, such as an alien invasion. Younger students could be directed to illustrate the school's fire drill in a poster format, using words and pictures.

Leading Questions:

1. Could this procedure be simplified?
2. Is it easily understood and followed by others?
3. How does it compare to the fire drill procedure?

Concept Formation

The students will discover that a planned response to an emergency is only helpful in a true emergency. They will find that if the school responded to non-emergencies as if they were true emergencies, it would be disruptive and annoying.

Leading questions:

1. What if the school really had an emergency that required this response?
2. What if the school decided to react this way every time the bell rang? whenever there was a power failure? whenever a stranger entered the building?
3. As more and more "threats" are added to the list, what happens?
4. Would the students and teachers take these situations seriously?
5. How much time could be potentially wasted?

Concept Application

The students will discuss their thoughts about the immune system's responses.

Leading question:

1. How does this compare to immune system reactions to threats in the human body?

Reactions

The students share their graphs and any discoveries they have made.

From *Serious Illness in the Classroom.* © 1997. Teacher Ideas Press. (800) 237-6124.

Emergency Plan

In case of _____

The alarm system will be _____

The plan for action is: _____

1. _____

2. _____

3. _____

4. _____

5. _____

These people are in charge of the following duties:

Person	Duty
_____	_____
_____	_____
_____	_____
_____	_____

On the back, draw a map that would assist your class, school, or town.

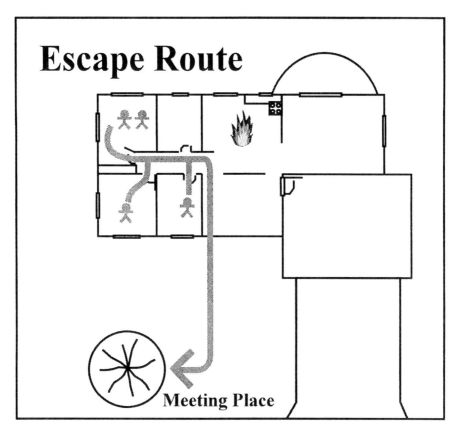

Example Fire Drill Map

Lesson 3 ━━━━━━━━━━━━━━━━━

Treatments and Precautions

Educational objectives:

1. To provide the students with information concerning how Allergies are treated and what precautions the patient must take.

2. To give students information necessary to enable them to assist a classmate with severe allergies.

Materials:

Three boxes, containing

1. the materials needed by the doctor to administer immunotherapy;

2. the emergency shot;

3. pictures or examples of Allergens that must be avoided.

Procedure:

1. Tell the students that each of the three boxes contains the materials used in the treatment of Allergies.

2. Tell the students to try and determine what the treatments in the boxes are by only asking questions that can be answered with replies of either yes or no. As the students gather data, they may ask the teacher for a "conference," during which they can review and discuss what they already know. The game resumes.

3. When they have discovered the answer, the box will be opened to allow the students to discover what the treatment entails and how it is used to help the person with Allergies.

4. After the boxes have been opened, list the three treatments on the board.

5. Have the different treatments explained and/or modeled by the school nurse, using the teacher as a model.

Closure

Divide the students into cooperative groups of two or three to create posters that will illustrate the treatments and precautions that have been modeled and discussed.

Lesson 4 ───────────────────────────

Vocabulary

Educational Objective

To provide students with opportunities to explore and understand vocabulary words associated with Allergies.

Word List

- Allergen
- Anaphylactic Shock
- Antibodies
- avoidance
- contagious
- digestive system
- immune system
- immunotherapy
- infections
- Respiratory system

Ideas for vocabulary activities:

1. Play a game of charades using the vocabulary words.

2. Create posters to illustrate the vocabulary using words and pictures.

3. Have students create a crossword puzzle using the vocabulary words.

4. Use the list as a substitute for a spelling list.

There are additional lesson ideas in the General Activities chapter.

Chapter 2

Asthma

Asthma is a noncontagious persistent lung problem that effects a person's ability to breathe by constricting air passages. Specifically, it impedes the lungs from fulfilling their basic purpose of removing carbon dioxide from the blood and replacing it with oxygen. Since Asthma does not usually go away, it is called a chronic respiratory condition. Children with asthmatic parents are believed to be more likely to have Asthma.

DESCRIPTION

The basic cause of Asthma is unknown. This condition is characterized by the constriction of the air passages from the nose and mouth to the lungs. This blockage results from either a sensitivity to triggers that causes narrowing of the airways, and/or increased mucus production that obstructs the airflow. As the air passages constrict, breathing becomes difficult, leading to wheezing, coughing, and/or shortness of breath. The blockage of the air passages caused by an asthmatic reaction is usually reversible either spontaneously or through the use of medication.

Asthma can develop at any age and the condition never disappears completely. Some asthmatics, however, may experience a decrease in the appearance of symptoms as they grow older. Poorly controlled or chronic Asthma can eventually decrease the function of the lungs, potentially slowing development in children. Emotionally, children dealing with Asthma commonly experience anger, fear, inferiority, depression, or guilt.

When breathing is normal, air travels through the nose or mouth to the throat, then to the trachea, or windpipe, and finally, to the lungs. From there, the air enters the bronchi, a rootlike system that looks like an upside-down tree. The bronchi is made up of tubes that branch off into consistently smaller tubes. The oxygen and carbon monoxide exchange in the blood occurs in the smallest of these tubes, which are called the bronchioles.

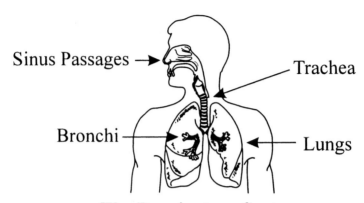

The Respiratory System

An Asthma attack mainly affects the bronchi. During an attack, the bronchial tubes swell, the surrounding muscles tighten, and mucus production increases. The swollen, mucus-clogged bronchial tubes restrict the airflow. It is difficult for the asthmatic to both inhale and exhale. Since not enough new oxygen arrives in the lungs, the oxygen level in the blood falls. These attacks are unpredictable and can last anywhere from a few minutes to several days. They can be life threatening. If, during an attack, the oxygen level falls very low, a dangerous condition called Cyanosis may occur. If the skin turns a purple-blue color—the main symptom of Cyanosis—medical help is necessary.

Asthma can damage the lungs, eventually causing them to lose their elasticity. This can lead to emphysema. Asthmatics are more susceptible to upper respiratory infections, such as bronchitis or pneumonia, because mucus secretions associated with Asthma do not always drain properly.

SYMPTOMS

The symptoms of an Asthma attack are easily observed. The asthmatic will be in obvious distress. Below is a short list of symptoms.

- coughing
- wheezing
- breathing difficulties
- chest tightness
- excess mucus

DIAGNOSIS

The diagnosis of Asthma is based on the child's medical history and the observable symptoms at the time of the evaluation. There are a number of tests that are used to confirm the initial diagnosis. Four common tests are spirometry/peak expiratory flow tests, chest X-rays, blood tests, and lung scans. In rare cases, sinus X-rays are used for diagnosis.

Common Tests

Spirometry/Peak expiratory flow test. This test monitors the lungs' function. It measures the amount of air that is inhaled and exhaled.

Chest X-rays. X-rays are used to create detailed pictures of the air passages and the various parts of the lungs.

Blood tests. These tests determine the amounts of the various substances in the blood.

Lung scans. Lung scans can create pictures of the whole lung or a specific part of the lung. These pictures accurately measure the lung's function. There are two different kinds of lung scans: the perfusion scan and the ventilation scan. The perfusion scan is more common and uses radioactive albumin, which is injected into a vein, to produce pictures of obstructions and lung functions. The ventilation scan is a test in which the patient breathes radioactive xenon gas while a scanner is passed over the lungs. It is used to show normal or abnormal bronchial passageways and areas of the lungs that do not receive air.

TREATMENT

The treatment of Asthma is designed specifically to meet the needs of each patient. Drug therapy is often a part of the treatment. There are medications that are used daily, and others that are used only during an attack. Several different types of medications are commonly used, including solutions, syrups, tablets, and inhalants.

Many asthmatics carry a small inhaler. Inhalers are potentially very dangerous. If they are not used correctly, they can even be fatal. The teacher and other supervising adults need to be aware of the proper use of the student's particular inhaler. This means that the directions for the use of the inhaler and the medication contained in its cartridge need to be given to the school. If the student's parents have not provided this information, school personnel need to request it. Usually, the inhaled medication takes about five minutes to take effect, and should relieve the symptoms for up to six hours. If the inhaler is needed more than four times in a full day, or twice during the school day, it may be a sign that the condition is deteriorating. Overuse of the inhaler is extremely dangerous. Consult the family, and if necessary, emergency medical personnel immediately if the child appears to be, or is obviously overusing her inhaler.

The most important step in treating Asthma is preventing an attack. Since treatments are individualized, it is necessary for the teacher and the school to become familiar with the specific needs of the students with Asthma. As the student becomes older, she needs to be allowed to be an active participant in her own care. The child must learn to read and respond to the early warning signs of an attack so that full-fledged attacks can be prevented.

WARNING SIGNS

 There are several different warning signs of an impending Asthma attack. These symptoms have been separated into early signs, general signs, and signs that demand immediate medical assistance.

Early Warning Signs

- pale, red, or swollen face
- irritability
- decrease in level of activity
- dark, under-eye circles
- excessive drooling

General Warning Signs

- changes in breathing (coughing, wheezing, breathing through the mouth, shortness of breath, breathing rapidly)
- tightness in the chest
- dry mouth
- neck pain or discomfort
- generally feeling ill
- change in normal behavior
- itchy chin or neck
- difficulty speaking

Dangerous Warning Signs

- chest pain
- an attack of severe proportions
- temperature of more than 100° F during an attack
- shortness of breath for no apparent reason

CLASSROOM CONSIDERATIONS

- avoid upholstered furniture
- vacuum and dust often
- use foam cushions
- choose class pets carefully—avoid warm-blooded animals
- avoid the child's particular triggers

COMMON TRIGGERS

- infections (colds, sore throats, bronchitis, tonsillitis)
- air pollutants (smoke, aerosols, perfumes, pollution, and cleaning agents)
- weather factors (cold air or high humidity)
- allergies (pollen, mold spores, animals, dust, food)
- emotional distress
- physical exertion
- exercise

CLASSROOM LESSON IDEAS

Lesson 1

What Is Asthma?

Educational Objective:

To introduce students to the term Asthma and its definition.

Materials:

Butcher paper set up as below.

K	W	L
What I Know	**What I Want to Know**	**What I Learned**

Procedure:

1. Begin the lesson by asking the class to brainstorm on what they already know about Asthma.

2. Fill out the "What I Know" section of the KWL chart with their suggestions.

3. Ask the students what their questions are concerning Asthma.

4. List these questions in the "What I Want to Know" section of the chart.

The next part of the lesson depends on the age of the students. Younger students can have their questions answered by the teacher, a visiting medical professional, or through a book read aloud to them. Older students may be given materials from which they can find the answers to their questions on their own. (This chapter on Asthma should be helpful.)

This activity can be conducted in cooperative learning groups or individually. After the students fill out their own "What I Learned" sections, the groups can reconvene and discuss their questions and answers. This ensures that the students draw correct conclusions about Asthma.

Closure

Discuss with the students why it might be important for them to know about Asthma, and how they can be supportive of a classmate with this condition.

Lesson 2 ───────────────

Lung Capacity

Educational objectives:

1. To illustrate the amount of air people use when inhaling and how much air they expel.
2. To develop the concept of the lungs and their purpose.

Expectations:

1. Students work within their groups.
2. Students speak at a whisper.
3. Students remain at their own tables.

Materials:

1. Large and small balloons.
2. Graphing materials.
3. Rulers.
4. Straws.
5. The lung diagram found at the end of this lesson.
6. The bronchiole diagram found at the end of this lesson.

Exploration Phase

Large and small balloons, straws, and rulers are given to the groups of students working together. Students are told to use these materials to measure the air they use when breathing in and the air they expel when breathing out.

Leading questions:

1. How can the balloon be used to measure the air we breathe?
2. What is the difference between the size of the balloon you are able to blow up in one breath and that of your partners?
3. Is it a good or a bad sign to be able to blow up a large balloon? Why?

Concept Formation

The students will discover that the ability to inflate a larger balloon suggests a larger lung capacity. They will discover that different people have different lung capacities. They will graph their lung capacity against that of their partners.

Leading question:

1. What would be the advantages or disadvantages of greater or lesser lung capacity?

Concept Application

The students will use the knowledge they gained to consider the damage Asthma can cause to the lungs and the effect the condition has on a person's ability to breathe.

Leading questions:

1. If Asthma causes lung deterioration, what happens to the amount of air used?

2. If only a small amount of air can be drawn into the body, what happens to that body?

The Lungs

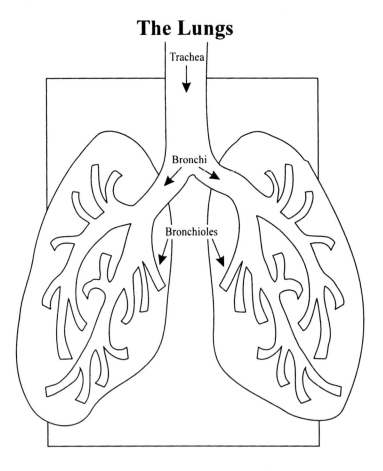

The Bronchioles

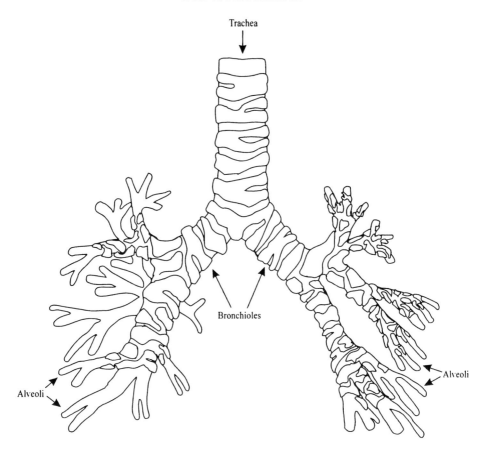

Lesson 3 ————————————————

Treatments and Precautions

Educational objectives:

1. To provide the students with information concerning the treatment of Asthma, and what precautions the patient must take.

2. To give students information necessary to enable them to assist a classmate with Asthma.

Materials

Three boxes, containing:

1. An inhaler.

2. Other Asthma medications.

3. Pictures of possible triggers that must be avoided.

Procedure:

1. Tell the students that each of the three boxes contains the materials used in the treatment of Asthma.

2. Tell the students to try and determine what the treatments in the boxes are by asking questions that can be answered with replies of either yes or no. As the students gather data, they may ask the teacher for a "conference," during which they can review and discuss what they already know. The game resumes.

3. When they have discovered the answer, the box will be opened to discover what the treatment entails, and how it is used to help the person with Asthma.

4. After the boxes have been opened, list the three treatments on the board.

5. Have the different treatments explained and/or modeled by the school nurse, using the teacher as a model.

Closure

Divide the students into cooperative groups of two or three to create posters that will illustrate the treatments and precautions that have been modeled and discussed.

Lesson 4 ——————————————————

Vocabulary

Educational Objective

To provide students with opportunities to explore and understand vocabulary words associated with Asthma.

Word List

- Allergies
- Asthma
- bronchial tree
- chronic
- contagious
- Cyanosis
- inhaler
- mucus
- reaction
- spirometry/peak expiratory flow test
- trachea
- triggers

Ideas for vocabulary activities:

1. Play a game of charades using the vocabulary words.
2. Create posters to illustrate the vocabulary using words and pictures.
3. Have students create a crossword puzzle using the vocabulary words.
4. Use the list as a substitute for a spelling list.

There are additional lesson ideas in the General Activities chapter.

Chapter 3
Cancer

Cancer is the common name for over 100 different non-contagious diseases. All of these diseases involve abnormal growth of body cells that tend to invade body functions and are capable of spreading to other parts of the body. Usually, cells divide and reproduce at a rate that enables growth, repair, and the necessary body tissue replacement. When cell growth gets out of control and divides more than necessary, the excess tissue forms masses. These masses are called tumors. Tumors that interfere with the functions of the body but do not spread to other locations in the body are known as benign, or noncancerous, tumors. Other tumors not only invade and destroy body tissue, but also break away from the original mass and spread to other parts of the body through the bloodstream or lymphatic system. This spreading is called metastasis, and this type of tumor is described as malignant, or cancerous. Both kinds of tumors are potentially harmful. They can invade and destroy normal tissue, and they deprive normal cells of nourishment and space. The five categories of cancerous diseases that will be addressed are: Leukemia, Lymphoma, Neuroblatoma, Brain Cancer, and Osteosarcoma.

DESCRIPTION

Although there are other types of cancer, some cancers are more common in children. The following are descriptions of the types of cancers that typically afflict children.

Leukemia

Leukemia is a cancer of the organs that make the blood: the bone marrow and lymph system. It is a cancer in which the bone marrow production of white blood cells is abnormal. In rare cases, the red blood cells are affected. Bone marrow is soft, fatty tissue found in the hollows of bones. It produces all of the red blood cells (erythrocytes), most of the white blood cells (leukocytes), and all of the platelets (thrombocytes). Normally, worn-out blood cells are replaced by new, mature blood cells, which fight infection. Leukemia causes white blood cells to enter the blood prematurely. These immature white blood cells, which flood the bloodstream, can not effectively fight off infections. People with Leukemia produce a large number of these immature white blood cells. Because the marrow is so busy producing white blood cells, it is unable to produce enough of the properly functioning blood cells that the body needs. It cannot produce enough healthy white blood cells to fight infection, enough red blood cells to carry an adequate amount of oxygen throughout the body, or enough platelets to control and prevent hemorrhaging. A person with Leukemia, therefore, is more likely to get infections and be unable to fight them off.

Lymphoma

Lymphoma is a cancer of the lymph system. The lymph system fights infections. It consists of a network of vessels that carry the lymph, a colorless liquid, throughout the body and to the tissues and organs that produce and store the white blood cells that fight infections. Lymphoma can spread to the bone marrow, liver, lungs, and bones.

Neuroblastoma

Neuroblastoma is a cancer of the sympathetic nervous system. This system regulates tissues such as the glands, muscles, and heart. The cancer is made up of immature nerve cells. They are usually found in the abdomen, but can also be found elsewhere in the body. Neuroblastoma can spread to the bone, bone marrow, liver, and the lymph nodes.

Brain Cancer

There are many different types of brain tumors, not all of which are cancerous. While a benign brain tumor does not spread to other parts of the body, it can still pose a problem. The skull cannot expand to accommodate a tumor growing inside. A malignant tumor can spread to other parts of the brain, the spine, and the nervous system.

Osteosarcoma

Osteosarcoma, or a bone tumor, often occurs in the knee, upper leg, or upper arm. These tumors are referred to as solid tumors. This cancer usually arises in areas of rapid bone growth.

SYMPTOMS

 ## General Symptoms of Cancer

(From the American Cancer Society)

- unusual bleeding or discharge
- a lump that does not go away
- a sore that does not heal within 2 weeks
- a change in bowel or bladder habits
- persistent hoarseness or cough
- indigestion or difficulty in swallowing
- change in a wart or mole

Symptoms of Specific Types of Cancer

Leukemia. Early symptoms of Leukemia are similar to those of a cold or the flu. The child may have a fever, suffer from loss of energy and appetite, and appear pale. In addition, there may be swelling of the lymph nodes, spleen, and liver; pain in bones or joints; a tendency to bleed or bruise; and frequent infections.

Lymphoma. The earliest sign of Lymphomas may be glandular swelling. The swelling usually occurs in the neck, armpit, or groin. Weakness, sweating, fever, nausea, vomiting, and itching may also occur.

Neuroblastoma. At the time of diagnosis, most children have lost weight; are cranky; lack interest; suffer from diarrhea, fevers, and abdominal pain; and have a slow rate of growth.

Brain cancer. The symptoms of brain cancer can vary greatly depending on the location of the tumor in the brain. Some common symptoms are changes in personality, memory, intellectual performance, and fine motor skills. Brain tumors can also affect vision and gross motor skills, and cause headaches, dizziness, nausea, and vomiting.

Osteosarcoma. The main symptoms of osteosarcoma (bone cancer) are swelling, pain, stiffness, tenderness, and difficulty using the affected body part. Osteosarcoma can also cause fractures, called pathologic fractures.

DIAGNOSIS

 The diagnosis of cancer begins with a complete medical history of the patient. This will include questions about his general health and the family history of cancer. Then many tests are conducted to determine if evidence of cancer is present. Some of these tests are described below.

Angiography

An Angiography is used to examine the blood or lymph vessels leading to the area of concern and it's blood distribution. The test uses X-rays to view these systems. A dye is injected into an artery or lymph vessel. This dye shows up in X-ray images. The X-rays, or angiograms, show the blood and lymph vessels and anything that is blocking these vessels.

Biopsy

A Biopsy is the examination of body tissue under a microscope. With this test, the examiner can detect and determine types of cancers.

Blood Tests

Blood tests are used to measure the number of white blood cells, red blood cells, platelets, and other substances in the blood. They are also used to locate and measure the amount of tumor markers. These are substances that are found in abnormal amounts when cancer is present.

Bone Marrow Aspiration

Bone Marrow Aspiration, or a bone tap, is used to check for cancer cells in bone marrow. A core of marrow is removed using a needle that has been inserted through the skin and into the center of the bone. This sample is examined for evidence of Leukemia.

Computed Tomography

Computed Tomography, or CT scan, produces detailed pictures of a suspected cancerous area. A number of X-rays are taken from a variety of angles. The information is coordinated to create a complete cross-sectional picture of the body. The picture allows for an accurate placement of a tumor(s).

Magnetic Resonance Imaging

Magnetic Resonance Imaging (MRI) uses powerful electromagnets, radio frequency waves, and a computer to produce an internal picture of the body. It is often used to diagnose brain tumors.

Radionuclide Scans

Radionuclide Scans use a small amount of radioactive material to examine various organs in the body. The radioactive substances are either swallowed by or injected into the patient. They then concentrate in areas of rapid cell division (a common sign of cancer). A scan is taken of the material, and its image displayed on a screen. This procedure is used to find cancers of the bone, kidneys, and other organs.

Ultrasound

Ultrasound uses very high frequency sound waves that bounce off inner bodily structures, leaving echoes of these structures behind. A picture of the inside of the body is created using these echoes. Tumors can be located using these pictures.

X-rays

X-rays are high energy electromagnetic waves that penetrate the body and produce pictures. These pictures are used to verify the presence and location of tumors.

TREATMENT

 There are three basic treatments for cancer: surgery, radiation therapy, and chemotherapy. A combination of these treatments is often used to fight cancer. New technology has enabled a more accurate diagnosis of this disease, which has allowed for an individual, and therefore, safer, and more effective treatment.

Surgery

In surgery, usually the tumor and a small amount of tissue that surrounds it are removed so that doctors can test for signs of cancer. Surgery is not used to remove all the cancer, but to see if any other treatment is necessary. If the cancer has spread, then treatments are needed. Surgery is most effective for the treatment of benign tumors.

Radiation Therapy

Radiation Therapy is the use of high-energy penetrating rays (subatomic particles) to either treat or control the cancer. Radiation injures the cancer cells' ability to multiply. This is administered at a dosage that does the least amount of damage possible to other cells of the body.

Chemotherapy

Chemotherapy treats cancer through the use of anticancer drugs. These highly toxic medications destroy cancer cells by altering their ability to grow and reproduce. Because the drugs are most destructive to cells that are dividing, they cause more damage to cancer cells than to other cells. The treatment must be carefully monitored, so that the dosage will kill the cancer cells without destroying too many healthy cells.

Another treatment occasionally used in Leukemia cases is bone marrow transplantation.

Bone Marrow Transplantation

Bone Marrow Transplants (BMT) replace damaged marrow with healthy bone marrow. Before the transplant can take place, the patient must undergo intensive radiation therapy and chemotherapy in order to destroy the cancer, as well as the remaining bone marrow. This is very dangerous, since without bone marrow, the patient is left completely unable to fight off infections. Its worth lies in the fact that this procedure makes it possible for donated bone marrow to be injected into the bloodstream and travel to the bones without confronting the threat of the cancer or the immune system's defenses.

Bone marrow transplants have the potential of being very successful in the treatment of Leukemia. However, these procedures are uncommon because it is difficult to find a matching donor for the patient. Typically, a close relative is the best donor candidate.

WARNING SIGNS

While there are warning signs in children before they are diagnosed with cancer, the teacher will probably only notice that the child is often not feeling well. After diagnosis, however, there are several things that a teacher should watch for. If any of these symptoms arise in the child, the parents, doctors, or emergency personnel should be notified immediately.

- infections
- bleeding
- headaches
- fever
- vision problems
- irritability
- sleepiness
- light sensitivity
- stiffness
- vomiting
- swelling or redness

SIDE EFFECTS

The treatment of cancer usually causes secondary, and undesirable, side effects. They are often harmful and painful. Each of the medications that is used to combat cancer has a different list of side effects. For example, patients treated with chemotherapy typically exhibit nausea, vomiting, and hair loss. The teacher should request the name of each medication with which the student is currently being treated, as well as the possible side effects from which the child may suffer. While the child may suffer the most from physical illness caused by treatment, the teacher may end up dealing with the emotional and social aspects related to the hair loss more than any other side effect.

INFECTIONS

Infections are dangerous to people who are fighting cancer. If a child on chemotherapy should come into contact with any infection, the parents and/or medical personnel should be notified. Exposure (even indirectly) to chicken pox or shingles can be fatal. Notification of such exposures must be made immediately.

AN EASY PRECAUTION

Start or reinforce a program of handwashing with soap in your school. If all students and school personnel consciously wash with soap a few times throughout the school day, the potential risks to the student with cancer are greatly reduced.

CLASSROOM LESSON IDEAS

Lesson 1

What Is Cancer?

Educational Objective:

To introduce students to the term cancer and its definition.

Materials:

Butcher paper set up as below.

K	W	L
What I Know	**What I Want to Know**	**What I Learned**

Procedure:

1. Begin the lesson by asking the class to brainstorm on what they already know about cancer.

2. Fill out the "What I Know" section of the KWL chart with their suggestions.

3. Ask the students what their questions are concerning cancer.

4. List these questions in the "What I Want to Know" section of the chart.

The next part of the lesson depends on the age of the students. Younger students can have their questions answered by the teacher, a visiting medical professional, or through a book read aloud to them. Older students may be given materials from which they can find the answers to their questions on their own. (This chapter on cancer should be helpful.)

This activity can be conducted in cooperative learning groups or individually. After the students fill out their own "What I Learned" sections, the groups can reconvene and discuss their questions and answers. This ensures that the students draw correct conclusions about cancer.

Closure

Discuss with the students why it might be important for them to know about cancer, and how they can be supportive of a classmate with this illness.

From *Serious Illness in the Classroom.* © 1997. Teacher Ideas Press. (800) 237-6124.

Lesson 2

What Is Metastasis?

Educational objectives:

1. To illustrate how cancer cells metastasize.
2. To allow the children to learn the definition of metastasis.

Expectations:

1. Students work in a safe manner.
2. Students speak at a whisper.
3. Students remain at their own tables.
4. Students follow the rules of the lesson.

Materials:

1. Cups.
2. A variety of individually wrapped candy.
3. Radio or tape deck and cassette tape.

Exploration Phase

Tell the students that this is a musical candy game. Have students wash hands first. Give them each five pieces of the same candy. (But vary the candy with each child.) Place a cup in front of each student with one of their kind of candies in it. Explain that the cups are to be passed along until the music stops. At each stop, students are allowed to trade one piece of their own candy for one piece of candy from the cup that ends up in front of them. (They are not allowed to eat the candy yet.) After a few rounds, have the students at each table discuss what happened to the candy.

Leading questions:

1. How much of your original candy do you still have?
2. Is there anyone who still has all of their original candy?
3. Does anyone have all new candy?

Concept Formation

Suggest to the students that they think about what this would mean if one of the types of candy was a germ. Have them discuss this. The students will realize that germs can transfer from one person to another.

Leading questions:

1. What would happen if one of the types of candy was actually a germ?

2. How could you explain how the germ moved around the table?

Concept Application

The students will discover that this is similar to the way that cancer cells travel throughout the body.

Leading questions:

1. What if the cups were actually the bloodstream within the body, that each student was an organ in the body, and that one type of candy was cancer?

2. Can you describe what the cancer would have done inside the body?

Explain that this transfer of cancer cells is called metastasis.

Reactions

The students share their discoveries.

Lesson 3

What Happens in the Bone Marrow of Someone with Leukemia?

Educational objectives:

1. To illustrate how bone marrow works.
2. To allow the children to discover how bone marrow is ineffective in a Leukemia patient.

Expectations:

1. Students work in a safe manner.
2. Students speak at a whisper.
3. Students remain at their own tables.

Materials:

1. Graph paper.
2. Scissors.
3. Crayons, markers, or colored pencils.
4. Glue.
5. Construction or butcher paper.
6. The bone marrow diagram at the end of this lesson.

Exploration Phase

Tell the students that their task is to make small, perfectly colored squares out of a piece of graph paper. (For older students, include the concept of area.) Explain that they must cover a larger piece of paper (construction or butcher) with the squares, creating a mural.

Leading Questions:

1. How many squares do you think you could make in five minutes?
2. How much effort does it take to make the squares perfect?
3. How long will it take your group to create the mural?

Concept Formation

The students will realize that they were forced to make shabby, unfinished squares that do not adequately cover the mural.

Quietly take the students' tools away from them. Tell them they must still attempt to create squares and cover the mural. Tell the students they have only five minutes to finish their murals, and that they MUST cover the mural in that time. They should be forced to scribble and tear out their squares.

Leading questions:

1. What will you do if I take away your scissors? and most of your crayons?

2. How much harder is it to make the squares?

Concept Application

The students will discover that they were forced to turn out inadequate squares. Relate this knowledge to what the bone marrow is forced to do in people with Leukemia.

Leading questions:

1. What happened?

2. Why did it happen?

Reactions

The students share their discoveries.

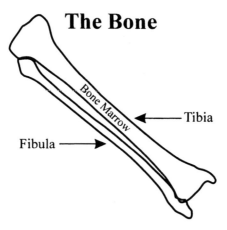

The Bone

Lesson 4 —————————————————————

Treatments and Precautions

Educational objectives:
1. To provide the students with information concerning how cancer is treated and what precautions the patient must take.

2. To give students information necessary to enable them to assist a classmate with cancer.

Materials:
Five boxes, containing
1. examples (either real or photographs) of the various tools used in surgery;

2. soap and a towel;

3. the materials needed by the doctor to administer chemotherapy;

4. the materials needed to administer radiation therapy;

5. the materials needed for a bone marrow transplantation.

Procedure:
1. Tell the students that each of the five boxes contains the materials used in the treatment of cancer.

2. Tell the students to try and determine what the treatments in the boxes are by asking only questions that can be answered with replies of either yes or no. As the students gather data, they may ask the teacher for a "conference," during which they can review and discuss what they already know. The game resumes.

3. When they have discovered the answer, the box will be opened to allow the students to discover what the treatment entails, and how it is used to help the person with cancer.

4. After the boxes have been opened, list the five treatments on the board.

5. Have the different treatments explained and/or modeled by the school nurse, using the teacher as a model.

Closure
Divide the students into cooperative groups of two or three to create posters that will illustrate the treatments and precautions that have been modeled and discussed.

Lesson 5 ──────────────

Vocabulary

Educational Objective

To provide students with opportunities to explore and understand vocabulary words associated with cancer.

Word List

- abnormal
- benign
- bone marrow
- contagious
- erythrocytes (red blood cells)
- glands
- immature
- infection
- invade
- Leukemia
- leukocytes (white blood cells)
- Lymphoma
- lymph system
- malignant
- mature
- metastasis
- Neuroblastoma
- Osteosarcoma
- thrombocytes (platelets)
- tumors

Ideas for vocabulary activities:

1. Play a game of charades using the vocabulary words.
2. Create posters to illustrate the vocabulary using words and pictures.
3. Have students create a crossword puzzle using the vocabulary words.
4. Use the list as a substitute for a spelling list.

There are additional lesson ideas in the General Activities chapter.

Chapter 4

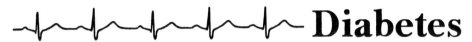 **Diabetes**

Diabetes is a disease in which the body is unable to process sugar due to a lack of insulin, a hormone produced by the body. There are two different types of Diabetes: Juvenile and Adult Onset. Children most often suffer from Juvenile Diabetes, which is also known as Type 1 or Insulin Dependent Diabetes.

DESCRIPTION

 Juvenile Diabetes is a disease in which the body does not produce enough insulin. Insulin is naturally produced by the pancreas, an organ found next to the gall bladder.

Pancreas

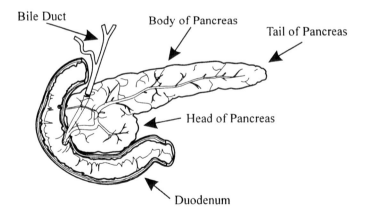

The pancreas releases the hormone directly into the bloodstream. Insulin helps sugar pass from the bloodstream into the body's cells, where it is burned for energy. Since Type 1 diabetics do not produce enough insulin, sugar cannot get to the cells. Instead, it stays in the bloodstream and builds up in the liver.

The sugar remaining in the bloodstream is treated as waste by the body. The kidneys are the organs that remove waste from the blood.

The Kidneys and Bladder

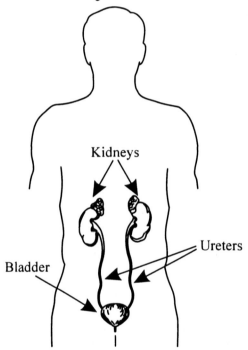

Waste from the blood is sent out of the body through the urine. The urine of untreated diabetics can be very high in sugar. The kidneys are overworked by the excess sugar which can cause severe complications with, or damage to, these organs. If the kidneys fail, the child with Diabetes must go on dialysis, a procedure that involves the use of a machine that removes the waste from the blood. If possible, there will be a kidney transplant. A transplant replaces the failed kidneys with at least one healthy kidney.

Juvenile Diabetes primarily occurs in children and young adults. However, it can happen at any age and is a gradual process. Although the cause of Diabetes is unknown, allergies, genetics, and the environment are three factors that are thought to be contributors to its onset.

SYMPTOMS

Several symptoms or combinations of symptoms often signal the onset of Type 1 Diabetes. These symptoms appear below.

- increase in urination
- extreme thirst
- hunger
- fatigue
- irritability
- weight loss
- stomachache
- vomiting
- blurry vision
- rapid breathing
- unconsciousness

DIAGNOSIS

If any of these symptoms persist in a child, it is important that the family seek medical attention in order to determine whether or not they suggest the onset of Diabetes. The doctor will administer blood and urine tests to determine if the patient has the disease. If the test results confirm Type 1 Diabetes, the doctor and family will begin the process of treating and controlling the disease. It is up to the medical staff to educate the family concerning their responsibilities in treating the child and on the impact Diabetes will have on the child's and the family's lives.

TREATMENT

Once Diabetes has been diagnosed, the treatment is tailored to the exact needs of the patient. A child with Diabetes, as well as her family, must become thoroughly knowledgeable about the disease and its treatment. Four important things a diabetic child should be made aware of in order to safely attend school are: how to administer blood and urine tests; how to administer insulin shots; her dietary restrictions; and how to recognize when she needs treatment for insulin shock.

Initially, a child with Diabetes will stay in the hospital where trained medical workers will develop a program for the patient and teach her how to take care of herself. The parents and child are taught how to take blood sugar tests, urine ketone tests, and how to administer insulin. To help understand the needs of the student with Diabetes, this information needs to be shared with the school so that the teacher can understand the tests. If necessary, a school official should ask for the information.

Blood Sugar Test

Blood Sugar Tests allow diabetics to more accurately control their blood sugar level. Blood sugar levels need to be monitored every day. The diabetic will be trained by medical professionals on what materials to use for the tests and how to properly administer them. The tests allow the diabetic to relate emotional and physical symptoms to blood sugar levels. They also provide the person with a sense of control over the disease and helps her to aim towards her ideal blood sugar level. The blood sugar test is highly effective because it provides immediate test results. This feedback enables the diabetic to understand the effects of various foods, exercise, and stress; to recognize a rapid fall in blood sugar; and if necessary, to adjust the dosage of insulin. These tests are, therefore, essential in the management of the illness.

Urine Ketone Test

The Urine Ketone Test is another very important aid for the diabetic. Urine ketones are chemicals that are produced when stored fat is broken down for energy. When not enough food is eaten to provide energy, ketones form in the blood. The ketones are later disposed of through the urine, where their presence can be detected by the Urine Ketone Test. The presence of ketones in the blood can result in stomach pain, vomiting, fast breathing, and frequent urination. This is called Ketoacidosis. Insulin and a healthy diet combat these symptoms.

Administering insulin prevents dehydration and Ketoacidosis. Diabetics are taught by their doctor how to give themselves insulin shots. Insulin can be injected in many places, and should be administered in a different part of the body every day. Two common places are the stomach and the thigh. As always, in a school setting such injections should be administered by the school nurse.

To prepare for the injection, the diabetic should carefully follow these steps:

- wash hands thoroughly with soap;
- warm and mix the insulin;
- clean the top of the insulin bottle with alcohol;
- measure the dose of insulin into the needle;
- clean the injection site with alcohol;
- pinch and hold the skin at the sight of injection;
- inject the insulin.

The diabetic must eat a healthy, well-balanced diet in order to successfully treat Diabetes, since food influences the blood sugar levels. The body also makes sugar, which adds to the level of sugar produced by food in the blood. The right amount and types of food are essential for good health. In general, the diabetic should eat food with fiber, starches, grains, fruits, and vegetables. Sugar and sweets, as well as salt and fat should be avoided. A person with Type 1 Diabetes should also maintain a healthy and appropriate weight and, in order to maintain a constant level of daily food intake, she should eat meals and snacks at the same time every day and use snacks to prevent insulin reactions. Excessive amounts of protein should be avoided.

At school, the student with Diabetes will require scheduled snacks and possibly an extra snack before P.E. There are many foods that are good schooltime snacks. Some of these foods are shown below.

- fresh or dried fruit and fruit juice
- popcorn
- nuts
- plain yogurt
- celery with peanut butter
- muffins, bread, crackers, and pretzels

Exercise is another key to maintaining the good health of a person with Diabetes. Blood sugar levels can be affected by exercise. It can help insulin work better in the body, and therefore, lower blood sugar. By increasing exercise, the diabetic can improve her health, maintain an ideal weight, lower the chance of heart disease, and lower her blood pressure.

At the present time, Diabetes is incurable, however, there have been recent reports of a discovery that may eventually lead to a potential cure for this disease.

WARNING SIGNS

There are several warning signs that signal the need for treatment in a person with Diabetes. They could indicate that the person's blood sugar level is either too high or too low. These signs are listed below.

- hunger
- shaking, sweating, and weakness
- glassy or dilated eyes
- pale or flushed face
- headaches
- drowsiness, inattention
- confusion, irritability, and personality changes
- speech changes
- unconsciousness

If a child's blood sugar is too low, the child may have

- forgotten to eat;
- not eaten all of a meal or snack;
- not eaten a meal or snack at the usual time;
- exercised more than usual;
- taken too much insulin.

If the blood sugar is too high, the child may have

- not taken enough insulin;
- eaten too much;
- exercised less than usual;
- taken ill.

CLASSROOM LESSON IDEAS

Lesson 1 ————————————————

What Is Diabetes?

Educational Objective:

To introduce students to the term Diabetes and its definition.

Materials:

Butcher paper set up as below

K	W	L
What I Know	**What I Want to Know**	**What I Learned**

Procedure:

1. Begin the lesson asking the class to brainstorm on what they already know about Diabetes.
2. Fill out the "What I Know" section of the KWL chart with their suggestions.
3. Ask the students what their questions are concerning Diabetes.
4. List these questions in the "What I Want to Know" section of the chart.

The next part of the lesson depends on the age of the students. Younger students can have their questions answered by the teacher, a visiting medical professional, or through a book read aloud to them. Older students may be given materials from which they can find the answers to their questions on their own. (This chapter on Diabetes should be helpful.)

This activity can be conducted in cooperative learning groups or individually. After the students fill out their own "What I Learned" sections, the groups can reconvene and discuss their questions and answers. This ensures that the students draw correct conclusions about Diabetes.

Closure

Discuss with the students why it might be important for them to know about Diabetes, and how they can be supportive of a classmate with this disease.

Lesson 2 ———————————————

An Insulin Bridge

Educational objectives:
1. To illustrate the idea that insulin acts as a bridge within the body.
2. To develop the concept of what a bridge does.
3. To use the idea of a bridge to teach students the role of insulin.

Materials:
1. Toothpicks or popsicle sticks.
2. Glue.
3. Cardboard for a base, if desired.
4. The Insulin Bridge diagram found at the end of this lesson.

Expectations:
1. Students work within their own groups.
2. Students speak at a whisper.
3. Students remain at their own tables.

Exploration Phase
Have the students build a bridge using the materials. Examples: drawbridge, suspension, or trestle.

Leading questions:
1. Are bridges necessities?
2. What are their uses?
3. Why would people want bridges?

Concept Formation
Students will discover that bridges are very useful and sometimes absolutely necessary.

Leading Questions:
1. When are bridges helpful?
2. Is there anything that can be used instead of a bridge to achieve the same purpose?
3. What are situations that require a bridge?

Concept Application

Explain that insulin creates a bridge between the bloodstream and cells. Present the Insulin Bridge diagram as an overhead. Explain that sugar (the fuel for energy) uses these bridges to move from the blood to the cells. Use the overhead to illustrate how insulin acts as the bridge. Students will see the connection between real-life bridges and insulin.

Leading questions:

1. What happens if there is no bridge between the bloodstream and the cells?

2. If there is no other way for sugar to get to the cells, what will happen to the cells and the body?

Reactions

Students share their discoveries with the class.

THE INSULIN BRIDGE

NORMAL

DIABETES

Lesson 3 ─────────────────────────

Sugar: How It Affects the Body

This activity must be done with the help of a nurse or medical professional. If there are concerns about the implications of this activity, it can be changed so that only the teacher and nurse model this type of experiment.

Educational objectives:

1. To allow children to observe the effect sugar can have on the body.
2. To determine, as a group, snacks that are healthy and appropriate for a person with Diabetes, and to encourage students to apply this knowledge to their own dietary habits.
3. To present treats that will be healthy, appetizing, and beneficial to everyone in the classroom.

Materials:

1. An overhead transparency of the Blood Sugar Levels chart found at the end of this lesson.
2. A healthy snack low in sugar. (Suggestions may be found at the end of this lesson.)
3. A sugary snack.
4. Supplies to test blood sugar.
5. Graph paper.

Procedure:

1. Two hours before the blood testing, have two students (with parent's written permission) eat the snacks with different ingredients. All students may be allowed to snack, but only two need to participate in the blood testing. The student with Diabetes and the teacher could be the two participants, or permission may be obtained from two other students to take the blood test.
2. Administer a sugar test to determine the levels of sugar in the blood.
3. Graph the results of the tests and compare them, allowing the students to list reasons why the results would differ.
4. Using a transparency of the blood sugar levels, discuss the safe levels for blood sugar, and determine whether the graphed results were within an acceptable range.

5. In groups of three or four, allow the students to
   a. discuss the importance of healthy snacks in the treatment of diabetes;
   b. cut pictures from magazines and make a collage of snacks that would be healthy for students with diabetes;
   c. make two or three healthy snacks to share with one another (recipes and ingredients provided by the teacher);
   d. compile a list of recipes to take home as healthy snack alternatives.

Closure

Have the students list two or three healthy snacks that could be kept in the classroom for the student with Diabetes. Determine an acceptable place for these to be stored in the classroom.

Snack suggestions:

- vegetables
- fruits
- celery with peanut butter
- crispy pretzels
- ginger snaps (made with molasses—no sugar)
- store-bought brownies or cookies for diabetics
- sugar-free candy
- sugarless gum

Blood Sugar Levels

RESULT	STATUS	SYMPTOMS
400-800	Very High	Stomach Pain Difficult Breathing
200-400	High	Little Energy
80-120 **DIABETIC TARGET RANGE** 100-200 80-180 70-150	Normal Up to 5yrs 5-12yrs 13 yrs and up	Fine
20-60	Low	Hunger Shakiness Sweating

Lesson 4 ——————————————

Treatments and Precautions

Educational objectives:

1. To provide the students with information concerning how Diabetes is treated and what precautions the patient must take.

2. To give students information necessary to enable them to assist a classmate with Diabetes.

Materials:

Four boxes, containing

1. the materials necessary to administer insulin;

2. the materials to measure sugar in the blood and urine;

3. several recipes for healthy snacks;

4. pictures of possible exercises, or a pair of running shoes.

Procedure:

1. Tell the students that each of the four boxes contains the materials used in the treatment of Diabetes.

2. Tell the students to try and determine what the treatments in the boxes are by asking only questions that can be answered with replies of either yes or no. As the students gather data, they may ask the teacher for a "conference," during which they can review and discuss what they already know. The game resumes.

3. When they have discovered the answer, the box will be opened to allow the students to discover what the treatment entails, and how it is used to help the person with Diabetes.

4. After the boxes have been opened, list the four treatments on the board.

5. Have the different treatments explained and/or modeled by the school nurse, using the teacher as a model.

Closure

Divide the students into cooperative groups of two or three to create posters that will illustrate the treatments and precautions that have been modeled and discussed.

Lesson 5 ————————————————

Vocabulary

Educational Objective

To provide students with opportunities to explore and understand vocabulary words associated with Diabetes.

Word List

- Blood Sugar Test
- dehydration
- Diabetes
- hormone
- insulin
- Ketoacidosis
- kidney
- pancreas
- Urine Ketone Test

Ideas for vocabulary activities:

1. Play a game of charades using the vocabulary words.
2. Create posters to illustrate the vocabulary using words and pictures.
3. Have students create a crossword puzzle using the vocabulary words.
4. Use the list as a substitute for a spelling list.

There are additional lesson ideas in the General Activities chapter.

Chapter 5
⎯⋀⎯⋀⎯⋀⎯⋀⎯⋀⎯ HIV/AIDS

Acquired Immune Deficiency Syndrome, or AIDS, is caused by a virus known as the Human Immunodeficiency Virus, or HIV. It attacks the body's white blood cells, eventually destroying the immune system. When this virus has taken its toll, the body is said to be immunodeficient. This means that its defenses have been weakened. By the time a person is diagnosed with AIDS, the body's defense system is either very weak or ineffective. After the virus has completely destroyed the immune system, a person is said to suffer from full blown AIDS.

DESCRIPTION

 HIV attacks and eventually destroys the body's immune system. This destruction occurs because the virus attacks T-cell lymphocytes, often called T-cells. T-cells are crucial to the body's defenses. They help fight off infections. HIV invades healthy T-cells by adding its own genetic material into the cell and becoming a permanent part of its genetic material. Later, when the T-cell reproduces, it will also produce more of the HIV virus. Because HIV is capable of changing its genetic material in order to become part of the genetic makeup of the cell it invades, it is called a retrovirus. Mild symptoms of HIV commonly appear a few years after the initial infection. These symptoms include fever, chills, sweats, fatigue, weight loss, diarrhea, and swollen lymph nodes.

At first, the body defends itself against the HIV virus. The immune system produces antibodies, chemical agents that locate and attack infecting organisms; in this case, the HIV virus. HIV, however, has the ability to alter itself in order to be unrecognizable to the antibodies. It does this by changing its outer coating.

Eventually, HIV destroys so many T-cells, that the immune system can no longer function effectively. The body is then a perfect environment for infections and diseases that would otherwise be easily fought off by a healthy immune system. These are called opportunistic infections. Opportunistic infections must be present before a diagnosis of AIDS can be made. Once the body has been infected with HIV, it becomes less and less able to fight off any infection until, eventually, one or more of them prove fatal.

HIV is transmitted, or caught, only through the exchange of bodily fluids. The virus lives in certain bodily fluids and secretions, especially blood and semen. Children can contract HIV from their mother before birth, or at the time of delivery. Although it is rare, they can also contract HIV from sexual contact or through the sharing of needles. Blood transfusions have been the cause of the transfer of the disease in the past, but because of positive changes in the control and safety of the blood supply in the United States this is no longer considered a threat. There have been no instances of children spreading HIV to others. Therefore, in a school setting, a child with HIV poses no risk to their classmates. Casual contact, such as hugging, touching, breathing the same air, or kissing *is not* a means of transmission of the virus.

SYMPTOMS

 There are no symptoms of HIV until a few years after infection. These symptoms may appear sooner in children, since their immune systems have yet to completely develop. The virus can eventually cause damage to body organs, developmental delays, and the loss of acquired skills as well as compromising the immune system. There are also some more specific symptoms that school personnel should watch for in a child with HIV or AIDS. The teacher should immediately notify the parents and/or medical personnel if any of these symptoms are observed.

- fever, chills
- sweating
- fatigue
- weight loss
- diarrhea
- swollen glands
- loss of appetite

DIAGNOSIS

There are three basic stages of the disease caused by HIV. Each is defined through the symptoms of the infection. When a person is first infected with HIV, they show no apparent signs of the disease and are termed asymptomatic. This first stage of infection is referred to as the incubation period. When symptoms develop, the patient is called symptomatic, or pre-AIDS. This is the second stage. Full blown AIDS is the third stage of the disease. When the symptoms become more severe, and specific problems due to HIV appear, a diagnosis of AIDS is made.

The only way to diagnose that a person has been infected with HIV is to test for the presence of antibodies to HIV in the blood. Antibodies are body chemicals that are produced by white blood cells to defend against disease. The body of a person with HIV will produce antibodies to the virus. These antibodies are ineffective. Their presence, however, indicates that there is an HIV infection. The confirmed existence of HIV antibodies is called an HIV-positive result. Usually, a second test is performed to verify the diagnosis. Because the antibodies do not show up for six months after the initial infection, an HIV-negative result needs to be followed up at that time with more testing.

There are two tests that are commonly used to diagnose the HIV infection. These are the Enzyme-Linked Immunosorbant Assay (ELISA) test and the Western Blot Test.

Enzyme-Linked Immunosorbant Assay

ELISA is a test that uses agglutination, or the clumping together of cells, to detect the presence of antibodies. Basically, a substance known as an antigen is introduced into a sample of the patient's blood. This antigen is one that is known to stimulate the production of antibodies to the HIV virus. If those antibodies are present, the cells will clump together as a defensive reaction to the antigen.

Western Blot Test

The Western Blot Test is a method of testing using a form of electrophoresis. In other words, an electrical charge is applied to the proteins so that their migration can be observed. These proteins aid in maintaining a balance of chemicals and plasma in the blood. They provide nutrition to tissues, and carry substances such as hormones, vitamins, drugs, and enzymes throughout the body. The Western blot test can give an indication of the presence of abnormal proteins in the blood.

A diagnosis of AIDS is not made until after the HIV virus has virtually destroyed the immune system of the patient. There are several specific illnesses that take advantage of the HIV-damaged immune system. The appearance of one or more of these infections indicates that the immune system is deficient enough for a diagnosis of AIDS. The specific infections include recurrent bacterial infections or opportunistic infections, such as pneumocystis carinii pneumonia (wasting syndrome), lymphoid interstitial pneumonitis, progressive neurological disease (encephalopathy), or certain cancers (malignancies).

TREATMENT

There is no known cure for HIV/AIDS. There are, however, several antiviral drugs that can be used to slow down the HIV infection, and possibly prolong life. These are acyclovir, AZT (zidovudine and azidothymidine), and DDI (dideoxyinosine). New drugs to treat HIV/AIDS are being developed every day. In fact, medical advances are currently being developed to better help HIV/AIDS patients. However, the average patient does not have access to these experimental treatments. At this time, since there is no known cure for HIV/AIDS, most of the treatment revolves around controlling the opportunistic illnesses, and on making life as livable as possible.

Because HIV destroys the immune system, it is difficult to treat patients for the opportunistic infections. Their compromised immune systems cannot assist the treatment and are often further damaged by the treatment. Some common treatments for opportunistic infections include antibiotics, radiation treatments, and chemotherapy.

WARNING SIGNS

Children with HIV should receive immediate medical help for all illnesses. Call the family or doctor if the child has been exposed to anyone who has the chicken pox, shingles, or measles. The family or emergency personnel should also be contacted if any of the warning signs listed below occur.

- fever
- breathing difficulties
- discomfort, pain
- loss of appetite
- vomiting
- diarrhea
- rashes
- frequent nose bleeds, bruises

- pale color
- delayed or slow development
- change in level of activity, or ability

PROTECTING THE CHILD WITH HIV/AIDS

A child with HIV/AIDS is unable to fight off infections. It is, therefore, necessary to try to prevent the child from getting infections in the first place. There are a few things that can be done to help keep the child's environment safe. First, every member of the school's population should be encouraged to wash their hands often with soap. Second, the child with HIV/AIDS should not only be encouraged but actively supervised to do the following while at school:

- wash hands with soap;
- eat nutritiously (including extra snacks);
- brush teeth after all meals;
- rest when necessary;
- use medications responsibly;
- use lotion to keep skin from drying and cracking;
- vocalize needs;
- behave normally.

INFECTIONS

Children who are HIV-positive are very vulnerable to other diseases. They are particularly prone to serious bacterial infections. These must be treated as soon as possible, usually with antibiotics, antifungals, and antivirals. The teacher needs to alert parents, and/or medical personal if signs of illness are noticed in the child. Since it is difficult to recognize many kinds of infections, the teacher should report all suspicions of illness. Some infections are listed below.

- blood infections
- ear infections
- intestinal infections
- meningitis
- oral thrush
- pneumonia
- skin infections
- urinary tract infections

These infections are dangerous for children with HIV/AIDS. The presence of these infections in the average child, however, does not mean that they have HIV/AIDS. These are infections from which healthy children also suffer.

CLASSROOM LESSON IDEAS

Lesson 1 ───────────────────────

What Is HIV/AIDS?

Educational Objective:

To introduce students to the terms HIV and AIDS and their definitions.

Materials Needed:

Butcher paper set up as below.

K	W	L
What I Know	**What I Want to Know**	**What I Learned**

Procedure:

1. Begin the lesson by asking the class to brainstorm on what they already know about HIV/AIDS.
2. Fill out the "What I Know" section of the KWL chart with their suggestions.
3. Ask the students what their questions are concerning HIV/AIDS.
4. List these questions in the "What I Want to Know" section of the chart.

The next part of the lesson depends on the age of the students. Younger students can have their questions answered by the teacher, a visiting medical professional, or through a book read aloud to them. Older students may be given materials from which they can find the answers to their questions on their own. (This chapter on HIV/AIDS should be helpful.)

This activity can be conducted in cooperative learning groups or individually. After the students fill out their own "What I Learned" sections, the groups can reconvene and discuss their questions and answers. This ensures that the students draw correct conclusions about HIV/AIDS.

Closure

Discuss with the students why it might be important for them to know about HIV/AIDS, and how they can be supportive of classmate with this disease.

Lesson 2 ———————————————

What Is a Retrovirus?

Definition: a retrovirus is a virus that is capable of altering the genetic material within a cell that it invades. It alters the genetic material so that when the host cell reproduces, it will also produce the virus.

Educational objectives:

1. To illustrate how a retrovirus works.

2. To help the children understand the definition of a retrovirus.

Materials:

1. Graph paper.

2. Scissors.

Expectations

1. Students work in a safe manner.

2. Students speak at a whisper.

3. Students remain at their own tables.

Exploration Phase

Tell the students that their task is to make perfectly measured squares out of a piece of graph paper. (For older students, include the concept of area.)

Leading questions:

1. How many squares do you think you could make in ten minutes?

2. How much effort does it take to make the squares perfect?

Concept Formation

The students will be tricked into making something other than what was actually needed.

Quietly suggest to the students that they may also make triangles as they make their squares.

Leading questions:

1. Do you think you could make some triangles as you make the squares?

2. How many would it be possible to make? Are you sure? Check and see.

Concept Application

The students will discover that they can be tricked just like the cells are tricked by HIV. They will relate this knowledge to the concept of a retrovirus.

Leading Questions

After a short time, ask the students to count the number of perfect squares that they were able to make. Write the names of the students, along with their numbers of squares, on the board. When the students ask for their triangle totals to be included, explain that you do not need any triangles. (They should be surprised.) Lead into a discussion about retroviruses.

Reactions

The students share their discoveries.

Lesson 3 ————————————————

Treatments and Precautions

Educational Objectives:

1. To provide the students with information concerning how HIV/AIDS is treated and what precautions the patient must take.

2. To give students information necessary to enable them to assist a classmate with HIV/AIDS.

Materials:

Three boxes, containing

1. examples (either real or photographs) of the various medications the HIV/AIDS patient may take;

2. soap and towels;

3. pictures depicting people who are sick with illnesses such as chicken pox, colds, and measles.

Procedure:

1. Tell the students that each of the three boxes contains the materials used in the treatment of HIV/AIDS.

2. Tell the students to try and determine what the treatments in the boxes are by asking only questions that can be answered with replies of either yes or no. As the students gather data, they may ask the teacher for a "conference," during which they can review and discuss what they already know. The game resumes.

3. When they have discovered the answer, the box will be opened to allow the students to discover what the treatment entails, and how it is used to help the person with HIV/AIDS.

4. After the boxes have been opened, list the three treatments on the board.

5. Have the different treatments explained and/or modeled by the school nurse, using the teacher as a model.

Closure

Divide the students into cooperative groups of two or three to create posters that will illustrate the treatments and precautions that have been modeled and discussed.

Lesson 4 ────────────────────

Vocabulary

Educational Objective

To provide students with opportunities to explore and understand vocabulary words associated with HIV/AIDS.

Word List

- Acquired Immune Deficiency Syndrome (AIDS)
- antibodies
- asymptomatic
- contagious
- fatal
- full blown AIDS
- genetic
- Human Immunodeficiency Virus (HIV)
- immune system
- immunodeficient
- infections
- opportunistic
- retrovirus
- semen
- symptomatic
- T-cells
- transmission

Ideas for vocabulary activities:

1. Play a game of charades using the vocabulary words.
2. Create posters to illustrate the vocabulary using words and pictures.
3. Have students create a crossword puzzle using the vocabulary words.
4. Use the list as a substitute for a spelling list.

There are additional lesson ideas in the General Activities Chapter.

Chapter 6

$\sim\hspace$ Serious Conditions in the Classroom

—————— EPILEPSY ——————

Epilepsy is a disorder of the central nervous system. It is the result of uncontrolled stimuli in the brain resulting in random or patterned muscular contractions, as well as other symptoms. It is a disorder, not a disease or mental illness. Epilepsy is not contagious. Epilepsy is characterized by sudden, recurring attacks, called seizures. The intensity of the seizures can vary from severe convulsions to a temporary lapse in awareness. Currently, there is no cure for epilepsy. Yet, various treatments have been quite successful. People with epilepsy are able to lead relatively normal lives.

DESCRIPTION

It is thought that epilepsy could be caused by heredity or genetics. At the very least, genetics may create a predisposition for epilepsy. When a person has a tendency to experience seizures, she is said to have epilepsy. Seizures are convulsions in which unconsciousness and even altered behavior occur. Epilepsy, or the tendency to have seizures, is usually caused by a burst of electrical energy in the brain. The burst is uncontrolled and short-term. Normal brain function involves constant controlled bursts of electrical energy. Life as we know it would not be possible if these bursts of energy did not occur. Epilepsy, or seizures, result when these normal electrical signals act abnormally by increasing or becoming erratic. Eighty percent of all diagnosed epileptics have no determined cause. Epilepsy is diagnosed by performing a test that enables doctors to study the brain's electrical activity.

67

The test is the electroencephalogram, often referred to as an EEG. There are three main categories of seizures; generalized, partial, and minor motor.

Generalized Seizures

Generalized seizures can manifest themselves in two forms. Many people have heard of these forms by their old names of grand mal and petit mal seizures. These types of seizures occur when the seizure involves most of the brain. In generalized convulsive seizures, historically called grand mals, all the muscles and motor functions of the body are affected by an abnormal burst of electrical energy. The person having the seizure will lose consciousness, fall, and go into convulsions that consist of the body stiffening and experiencing quick, jerky movements. The person may also lose control of the bladder and the bowel. A few minutes after the seizure, the person will usually regain consciousness but will be confused. She will usually feel tired and need rest. Soon, however, she should be able to rejoin the day's regular activities. These seizures usually last a few minutes and can be as common as once a day or as rare as once every two to three years.

Another type of generalized seizure is less dramatic and lasts only a few seconds. It involves a brief lapse in consciousness. To the untrained eye, this type of seizure can look similar to inattention or "spaciness" for a moment. A child will stop midsentence, stare for a moment, and then pick up as if there had been no break. The seizure can also consist of increased blinking or chewing, waving arms, and a turning head. These used to be called petit mal seizures but are now referred to as absences. The medical term is generalized nonconvulsive seizures. They can occur multiple times a day or just once or twice a month. They may be subtle and extremely hard to detect.

Partial Seizures

Another major category of seizure types is referred to as partial seizures. These involve the abnormal discharge of energy into only one part of the brain. They are sometimes referred to as temporal lobe or psychomotor seizures. Partial seizures are the most difficult to recognize. Sometimes the child will lapse into automatic behavior. She will go through the motions of something, but will remember none of it after the seizure. The automatic behavior could include a mimed conversation, sitting, standing, walking, or even a common chore.

Other partial seizures are called focal motor seizures. These seizures show up as sudden, jerky motions in only one part of the body. The child may also think she hears, sees, or tastes something that is not present. This is called a sensory hallucination. This can be extremely frightening for the child. The cause of these phantom sensations is the same electrical bursts in the brain that cause the other seizures. These seizures are often preceded by a sense of fear in the child.

Minor Motor Seizures

Minor motor seizures, or myoclonic epilepsy, is uncommon. It is found in very young children. This type involves an increased sensitivity, or hypersensitivity, to light. It is thought to be inherited.

IN THE CLASSROOM

Since seizures happen unexpectedly, it is safer for a child with epilepsy to be around people who are aware of the epilepsy and can help. Classmates need to be taught that epilepsy is a disorder that causes the brain to temporarily change. It can cause a blackout. A child may fall to the floor, shake all over, and become very stiff. Seizures can cause parts of a person's body to shake or make sudden movements. They can also cause stomach pain, anger, or fear. A child can appear sleepy or sluggish. She can walk around, going through the motions of life, but not make sense. A child having a seizure has no control over her body or actions. After a seizure the child will need reassurance that she is all right.

At school, a child experiencing a severe seizure can be helped to prevent injury. Objects surrounding the seizing child should be removed. Loosen tight clothing, especially around the neck, and saliva can be wiped away. If the child vomits during the seizure, she should be turned on her side so that the vomit is not swallowed or choked on.

There are many misconceptions about seizures that lead to numerous "don'ts" when dealing with a seizure. Do not attempt to restrain a seizing child in any way (unless, during a more moderate seizure, the child begins to wander into danger). Do not put anything in the child's mouth. It is not possible to swallow the tongue during a seizure. Do not try to snap the child out of the seizure by shaking, slapping, or throwing cold water. Most importantly, do not panic. The child does not feel pain during a seizure and will naturally turn blue or even stop breathing for a short time during a seizure. If possible, the teacher should try to observe the seizure closely. The medical personnel working with the child with epilepsy can use any information about a seizure that the teacher can report, such as the duration, part of body involved, and progression of symptoms.

If the seizure lasts for more than a few minutes (don't panic) the teacher needs to call 911 and then follow the school procedure for contacting the family.

Seizures can also be caused by high fevers, brain injury or infection, and drugs or poison. Most of these seizures are limited. They can be cured or will eventually go away. Epilepsy, however, is a life-long condition. A child with epilepsy will have seizures until a doctor is able to control them with treatment. The treatment usually consists of anticonvulsant drugs or tranquilizers. The result of the use of medications varies. Sometimes the seizures are prevented. Other times there is a reduction in the severity of the seizures. Surgery can be, but is rarely, used as treatment.

GRIEF

Grief is defined as deep mental anguish. It is the process of dealing with a profound loss. Children grieve just like adults. However, as children grieve, they are less likely to recognize all their feelings as part of their grieving. Grieving children need help to understand their feelings.

DESCRIPTION

Grief is the reaction to and then the process of recovering from the loss of someone or something that was loved. It is experienced after, and most often associated with, a death. It can also be experienced after a divorce—which represents the virtual loss of a parent—or because of a forced long-term separation—sometimes caused by a move. People usually go through many stages of grief. Each person, however, experiences each stage in a unique way. Many people experience anger, fear, disbelief, and various degrees of depression.

Grief is a highly personal experience. Often, the first stage is that of shock. Initially, a grieving person might feel dazed and does not seem to fully comprehend the loss. Once the child realizes what has occurred, a variety of emotions such as anger, guilt, resentment, anxiety, and despair commonly surface. As the person gradually accepts the loss, he begins to adjust to it. Eventually the loss is accepted. The goal is to work through the grieving process so that ultimately life can be looked at as a positive experience again instead of as a depressed state. Children often display their grief through their behavior. A grieving child can begin to look as an angry or a depressed child. He might begin to misbehave. Although acceptance is usually reached after two years, some children really do not begin to grieve until a year has passed after the death. They often appear to be handling the death of a loved one quite well. Yet as the anniversary date approaches, their grieving will intensify. Another difficult time for children, as well as adults, is the holidays.

IN THE CLASSROOM

Honesty is the only policy.

A grieving child needs to express himself. The teacher needs to be aware of a child's need to express emotions and the difficulty the child may have in finding an outlet and a method for that expression. Words, pictures, role playing—anything that works should be available. Since each individual child will grieve and express himself in a unique way, there is no recipe for success for dealing with the child. The teacher needs to be flexible yet aware of the possibilities. Open honesty is the best policy. The teacher should not refuse to talk about the loss nor should the teacher avoid accidentally mentioning the name of or referring to the deceased. This will only serve to remind and reinforce the idea that the teacher is uncomfortable and therefore unable or unwilling to help the child.

Communication is essential, even if it is extremely difficult for the adult. The child needs for the adult to put personal anxieties aside. Children need to be taught that their feelings are normal and okay. The teacher is in an excellent position to reinforce this.

School can essentially be a safe place for life to continue for the grieving child. At school, virtually nothing has changed. They are not constantly aware and reminded of their loss. (If the loss was that of a teacher or a classmate, then home is the safe place.) The child may choose or simply try to use school in this way, as a break from the pain. However, children, unlike adults, are usually unskilled at hiding their feelings. If they are feeling something, they usually express it in some way no matter where they are.

When the grieving becomes overwhelming for the child it will be apparent at school. The child's behavior usually will change. He may become artificially bright, depressed, angry, weepy, or exhibit any number of other emotions. The key is that there will be a change in the child's behavior. This change probably signals a need to process through another aspect of the loss or the grieving process.

Teachers who feel unable to deal with the potential needs of a grieving child need to ask for help from the appropriate school personnel. A child spends a major part of his waking hours at school. It is healthier for the child if there is an outlet for him during this time spent at school. At the very least, he should contact a family member if needed during school hours.

Children need to be led into a positive attitude, so that they feel like continuing on with life. It is possible that children might need to have extended assignment opportunities. Their life might not always allow for homework— and they might not be capable of concentrating all the time. The teacher should not hesitate to call upon the school's counseling resources.

HEMOPHILIA

Hemophilia is an inherited disorder characterized by excessive bleeding. It is not a disease and it is not contagious. At this time, there is no cure. There are, however, successful treatments.

DESCRIPTION

Hemophilia is the general name of several blood disorders in which the blood clotting process takes much longer than normal. People who have hemophilia have low levels of the substances that are responsible for coagulation, or clotting in the blood. There are fourteen steps in the process to halt bleeding. In hemophilia, one of the clotting steps is disrupted because of a lack of a protein, which is necessary to complete that step.

Hemophilia is a genetic disorder. This means that hemophilia is passed from parent to child, usually mother to son. Males are usually affected, while women are usually carriers, having inherited the gene from one of their parents, but not showing symptoms. Carriers are able to pass on the disorder or the genes to their children.

Although hemophilia can be diagnosed prenatally through blood sampling and DNA tests, many cases are not diagnosed until later. Symptoms usually begin to appear when the child first becomes active. Bruises are common in and around the joints. Because of internal bleeding into the joints, they are easily damaged and quite painful. Another symptom is excessive external bleeding. Minor injuries, such as scrapes and cuts, will cause an abnormal amount of blood loss. This, however, is not the greatest threat, or most serious symptom. Bleeding can occur spontaneously and is most apt to happen during times of rapid growth (5-15 years or K-9th grade). Internal bleeding can be identified through blood in the stool or urine, or through extensive bruising.

There are three forms of hemophilia known as hemophilia A, B, and C. Hemophilia A and hemophilia B are much more common than hemophilia C. Hemophilia A, the most common, is also called classic hemophilia. Hemophilia B is often referred to as Christmas disease because Stephen Christmas was one of the first patients with this disorder to be studied. The least common, hemophilia C, is seen most often in people of Ashkenazi Jewish decent. The hemophilias differ in the missing protein in the co-agulation process within the blood. A range in the level of clotting that hemophilia allows means that a person could have from mild to severe hemophilia.

Hemophilia is diagnosed through blood tests that look at the levels of the various clotting factors. Carriers of hemophilia can be identified through DNA analysis.

The treatment involves regular transfusions of the clotting factor that is missing in the blood of a person with hemophilia. If serious bleeding episodes occur, hospitalization is necessary. Some patient's immune system begins to attack the infusions by creating antibodies to fight the transfused clotting factor. This makes it very difficult to treat the patient. Luckily, not all immune systems react in this way. Severe cases of hemophilia require transfusions as often as once a week.

HIV/AIDS has been a real threat to people with hemophilia because of possible infection from tainted blood during transfusions. Today, however, it is believed that the blood supply in the United States is safe. Future transfusions should not jeopardize the health and life of people with hemophilia.

IN THE CLASSROOM

It is possible to lead a relatively normal life with hemophilia. However, it is necessary to attempt to avoid injury. At school, this means that rough play and some recess activities might have to be restricted. However, as most people who have spent time around children know, it is virtually impossible to completely protect children from getting hurt. The school personnel must be ready to meet the child's needs if an injury occurs. These needs can include the immediate cessation of activity, cleansing of wounds, and application of pressure. The bandages, or dressings, for wounds should be close at hand (in the classroom, and with the supervising adult at recess). Parents should be notified as soon as is possible in the event of an injury.

——————— SICKLE-CELL ANEMIA ———————

Sickle-cell anemia is characterized by the presence of oxygen-deficient red blood cells, episodes of pain, and leg ulcers. It is hereditary and is not contagious.

DESCRIPTION

The inherited blood disorder, sickle-cell anemia, is a chronic, or life-long, condition. It is the result of an abnormality within the red blood cells, the erythrocytes, that eventually deform the red blood cells. These red blood cells contain an abnormal type of hemoglobin called hemoglobin S. Normally, hemoglobin carries oxygen in the blood throughout the entire body to nourish body cells. Hemoglobin also provides the red color to the blood. Hemoglobin S is caused by an amino acid within the hemoglobin molecule. Hemoglobin S causes the red blood cells to collapse when there is a lack of oxygen in the cell. Normal red blood cells are round and flexible. When the red blood cells collapse, they have a crescent or sickle shape. Hence the name of the disorder. The sickled cells are inflexible and fragile. The red blood cells are most likely to collapse after they deliver the oxygen they are carrying and become oxygen deprived. They can break and tend to become entangled with each other and block blood vessels. When these cells have blocked a blood vessel, a vicious cycle begins. The lack of circulation causes an oxygen deficiency, which in turn causes more blood cells to sickle. When blood vessels become blocked, pain and damage occurs in the affected area. When organs are involved, the condition can be life threatening.

This condition most often affects African Americans, however, it can occur in any race. It only occurs when a child inherits the gene from both parents. If only one gene is inherited, the person is said to be a carrier and usually shows no symptoms of the condition. The severity of this disorder varies greatly. The life span, however, of a person with sickle-cell anemia is usually shortened.

At this time, there is no cure for sickle-cell anemia. Drugs to combat the sickling are being researched and tested. During a crisis, people with this condition are treated with painkillers, oxygen, and since dehydration can occur during a crisis, fluid intake and output is monitored. Diet and medication are used to prevent dehydration.

IN THE CLASSROOM

Visual symptoms of sickle-cell anemia are the same as other anemias. They include fatigue, quickened heart beat, and a feeling of breathlessness. A more serious symptom of sickle-cell anemia is referred to as a crisis (i.e., when the sickled cells block off the blood supply to vital areas of the body). People with sickle-cell are apt to experience painful and potentially life-threatening sickle-cell crises. Crises occur when the abnormal sickle-shaped red blood cells are unable to pass through small blood vessels. If the cells cause the vessel to become blocked, blood cannot circulate. If oxygen-rich blood is unable to circulate throughout the body, then the body is deprived of necessary oxygen. This can result in damage to tissue or even organs.

Other symptoms can include developmental delays, leg ulcers, vision problems, and organ damage. The spleen is often affected, leading to a compromised immune system. This can leave the person with sickle-cell anemia unable to effectively fight off infections.

Another concern that teachers need to be aware of is that a child with sickle-cell anemia is at risk when even a minor injury occurs. People with sickle-cell anemia do not have the ability to stop their blood flow through clotting because of the medication that they are usually taking to suppress the sickling of their red blood cells. This means that any injury that may cause bleeding—internally or externally—is dangerous. A student with sickle-cell anemia must be watched carefully if an injury has taken place. If there is any question of whether or not there may be internal bleeding, the school must contact medical personnel and the family of the student. This should also be done if external bleeding continues for a period longer than normal (as determined by the school nurse).

In case of external bleeding, the school needs to meet the safety needs of the child. These needs include the immediate cessation of activity, cleansing of wounds, and the application of pressure. Bandages, or dressings, should be close at hand (in the classroom and at recess with the supervising adult). Parents should be notified as soon as possible.

CLASSROOM LESSON IDEAS

Lesson 1 ————————————————

What Is This Condition?

Educational objective:

To introduce students to the condition and its definition.

Materials:

Butcher paper set up as below

K	W	L
What I Know	**What I Want to Know**	**What I Learned**

Procedure:

1. Begin the lesson by asking the class to brainstorm on what they already know about the condition.

2. Fill out the "What I Know" chart with their suggestions.

3. Ask the students what their questions are concerning the condition.

4. List these questions in the "What I Want to Know" section of the chart. The next part of the lesson depends on the age of the students. Younger students can have their questions answered by the teacher, a visiting medical professional, or through a book read aloud to them. Older students may be given materials from which they can find the answers to their questions on their own. (This chapter on conditions should be helpful.)

This activity can be conducted in cooperative learning groups or individually. After the students fill out their own "What I Learned" sections, the groups can reconvene and discuss their questions and answers. This ensures that the students draw correct conclusions about the condition.

Closure

Discuss with the students why it might be important for them to know about the condition, and how they can be supportive of their classmate.

Lesson 2

Vocabulary

Educational Objective

To provide students with opportunities to explore and understand vocabulary words associated with the condition.

Word Lists

Epilepsy

- central nervous system
- contagious
- convulsions
- disorder
- electroencephalogram (EEG)
- epilepsy
- generalized seizures
- genetic
- hereditary
- hypersensitivity
- inherited
- partial seizures
- seizures
- stimuli

Grief

- anger
- death
- depression
- grief
- profound
- sadness
- shock

Hemophilia

- clotting
- coagulation
- disorder
- external
- genetic
- hemophilia
- immune system
- inherited

- internal
- non-contagious
- transfusion

Sickle-cell Anemia
- chronic
- circulation
- crisis
- disorder
- fragile
- hemoglobin
- inflexible
- oxygen
- sickle-cell anemia
- ulcers

Ideas for vocabulary activities:
1. Play a game of charades using the vocabulary words.
2. Create posters to illustrate the vocabulary using words and pictures.
3. Have students create a crossword puzzle using the vocabulary words.
4. Use the list as a substitute for a spelling list.

MORE CLASSROOM IDEAS

Epilepsy

Lesson 1—Seizures

Objectives:

1. To familiarize the class with seizures.
2. To teach and practice the proper reaction to a seizure.
3. To increase the safety of the child with epilepsy at school.

Procedure:

Facilitate the role playing of a variety of situations in which a seizure takes place. Allow different students to play all of the roles, including that of the seizing child. Promote a calm, helpful attitude.

Closure

After using this to become familiar with the proper reaction to a seizure (seen earlier in this chapter), the class may want to add specific ideas that pertain to the school or classroom. The class could develop a specific procedure to share with other teachers and to provide to substitute teachers. (If this is not done by the students, the teacher should provide it.)

Lesson 2—A Bombardment

Educational Objectives:

1. To illustrate the idea of a burst of energy that over-stimulates the brain.
2. To develop the concept of this burst of energy.

Materials:

Choose between the following for each student.

1. Noisemakers.
2. Musical instruments.
3. Flashlights.
4. Colored pieces of paper.
5. Flags.

Expectations—If done as a small group

1. Only work within your group.
2. Whisper.
3. Stay in your workspace.

Exploration Phase

Have the students play with the material given to them. If this is in a large group situation, each student should have the same thing. In smaller groups, each member of a group should have the same thing.

Leading Questions:

1. What are some words you can use to describe what you have?
2. What could you use this for?

Ask one student to watch the other students as they calmly and slowly show the materials in the group. Do this with no talking. The student watching should then be asked to describe what was seen or heard.

Leading Questions:

1. Which person showed you their material first?
2. In what order did you see or hear things?
3. Was this confusing?
4. Can you describe everything that happened?

Concept Formation

Direct the students to speed up the process. Have them quickly (and often) flash their materials at the student watching.

Leading Questions:

Use the same as above.

Concept Application

Explain that this activity illustrates what happens within the brain when it is overstimulated.

GRIEF

Lesson 1—Active Listening

Educational Objectives:

1. To teach and practice the art of active listening.
2. To openly discuss grief and death.

Procedure:

1. Explain to the students that active listening involves listening so well that you can repeat and remember what you have heard. It also involves making sure that the person who is talking to you knows that you are listening.

2. Ask the students to brainstorm a list of actions that show through body language that a person is listening.

3. Together condense this list into a short list that can be posted in the classroom.

4. Model the art of responding to someone while repeating back some of what was said by asking a few students questions and then responding appropriately.

5. Ask for volunteers to try this with you.

The next steps can be done by the teacher or a school counselor.

6. Introduce the idea of death and grief.

7. Allow the students to discuss their thoughts and feelings openly.

8. Answer questions honestly.

9. Promote the use of actively listening.

Lesson 2—Ease Tensions

Objectives:

1. To allow students to work through their nervousness about the return of their classmate.

2. To develop the idea that the grieving child needs comfort but also needs to be treated normally.

Procedure:

Facilitate the role playing of a variety of situations in which different students may have initial contact with the grieving child. Discuss that the person who has died can be mentioned. Explain to students that their classmate may want to talk about the loss. Students, however, should listen carefully and try to follow the needs of the grieving child.

Hemophilia

Lesson 1—Following Directions

Educational Objectives:
1. To illustrate the idea that the process of blood clotting is a series of steps.
2. To develop the idea of a missing tool in the clotting process.

Materials:
1. Toothpicks or popsickle sticks.
2. Glue.
3. Rulers.
4. Crayons, markers, or paint.

Expectations:
1. Only work within your space.
2. Whisper.
3. Stay in you workspace.

Exploration Phase

After passing out the toothpicks (or popsickle sticks) and the coloring tools, quietly give each student (or group of students) only one of the other two materials (glue or a ruler). This means that each student will be missing a tool while they attempt to complete this activity. This may be frustrating for them—so prepare.

Direct the students to build something with specific dimensions.

Example: A box that is 3 inches by 3 inches.

When students complain that they cannot complete the assignment, ask them to either write down an explanation of why or, for younger students, have them explain orally.

Concept Formation

Ask the entire class to explain what the problem is. They should come up with something such as "There are tools that are needed missing." Lead them into a discussion about tools and needs within the body.

Concept Application

Share the fact that hemophilia involves missing tools within the blood. Explain that this means that the directions for clotting blood cannot be followed.

Gather up the materials or use this as a cooperative activity in which students have to share to finish the assignment.

Sickle-cell Anemia

Lesson 1—Oxygen Deprivation

Educational Objectives:

1. To illustrate the need for oxygen in living things.
2. To develop the concept of what happens inside the body when blood cannot circulate.

Materials:

1. A match and a candle.
2. An air-tight, see-through container (for the lit candle).
3. A small plant.
4. A plastic bag with a tie.

Procedure:

Explain to the class that fire needs oxygen to exist. Fire uses oxygen as energy. Also explain that the see-through container is air-tight. Demonstrate fire's need for oxygen by lighting the candle and then placing it inside the air-tight container. Have the students observe the candle's flame going out. Discuss the observations.

Now explain that plants and animals also need oxygen to survive. Demonstrate this using the plant and the plastic bag. Place the plant (or part of a larger plant) inside the bag and put it aside for a few days. Observe the plant later.

It might need to be emphasized that these are extreme examples. They do, however, illustrate why parts of the body protest their lack of oxygen through the pain that the person with sickle-cell anemia feels.

Have students share their discoveries with the class.

There are additional lesson ideas in the General Activities Chapter.

Chapter 7

⌐ᴠᴧᴠᴧ⌐ # General Activities

ACTIVITY 1

Learning About the Human Body

Educational objective:

1. To introduce an aspect of the human body

   a. Body systems and their purposes

      (1) Respiratory System—to obtain and use oxygen and eliminate carbon dioxide from the body

      (2) Skeletal System—to provide structure, strength, and mobility to the body

   b. The major organs of the body

   c. Ingredients of the blood

Materials:

The informational diagrams on the following pages.
Ideas for uses:

- memory lesson
- visual aid
- research starting point
- coloring sheet

Name _____ Date _____

The Respiratory System

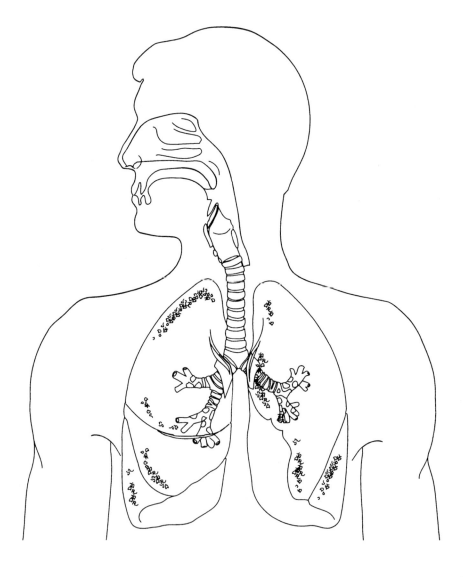

Name _____ **Date** _____

The Respiratory System

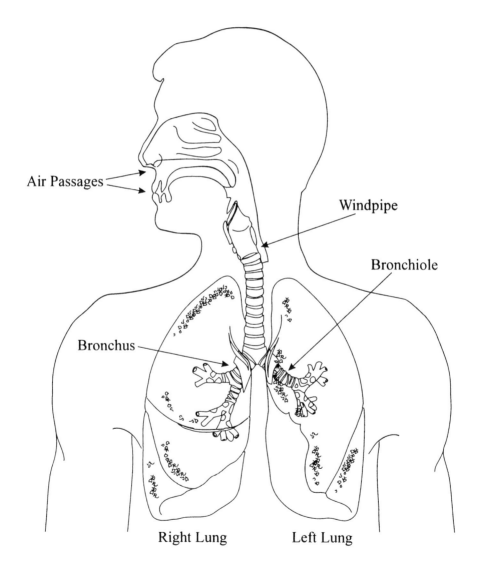

Air Passages

Windpipe

Bronchiole

Bronchus

Right Lung

Left Lung

Name ————————————————— Date ———————

The Skeletal System

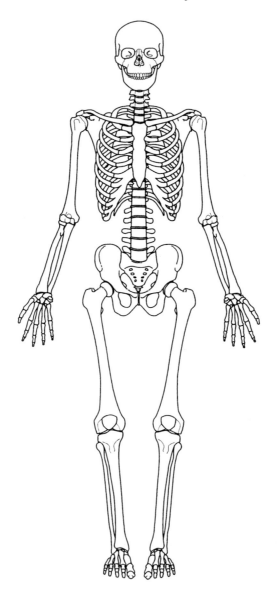

Name ——————————————— **Date** ———————————

The Skeletal System

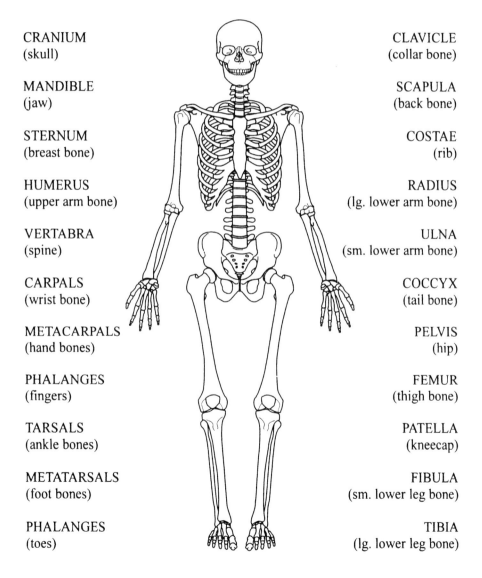

CRANIUM
(skull)

MANDIBLE
(jaw)

STERNUM
(breast bone)

HUMERUS
(upper arm bone)

VERTABRA
(spine)

CARPALS
(wrist bone)

METACARPALS
(hand bones)

PHALANGES
(fingers)

TARSALS
(ankle bones)

METATARSALS
(foot bones)

PHALANGES
(toes)

CLAVICLE
(collar bone)

SCAPULA
(back bone)

COSTAE
(rib)

RADIUS
(lg. lower arm bone)

ULNA
(sm. lower arm bone)

COCCYX
(tail bone)

PELVIS
(hip)

FEMUR
(thigh bone)

PATELLA
(kneecap)

FIBULA
(sm. lower leg bone)

TIBIA
(lg. lower leg bone)

Name ——————————————————— Date ——————————

The Major Organs of the Human Body

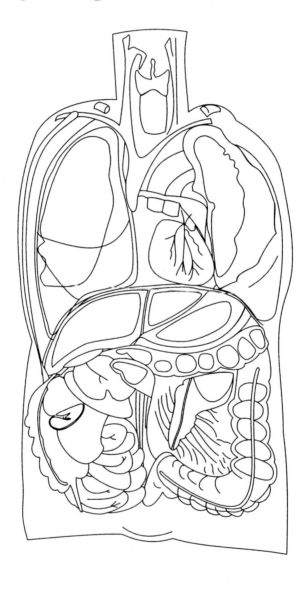

Name ——————————————— Date —————————

The Major Organs of the Human Body

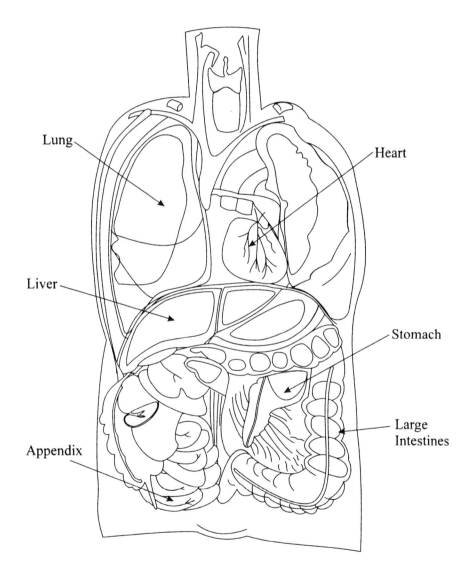

Lung

Heart

Liver

Stomach

Large
Intestines

Appendix

ACTIVITY 2

The Importance of Washing Your Hands

Educational Objective:

To explain and illustrate the necessity of cleanliness when fighting germs.

Materials:

1. Different colored stickers.
2. Two to three poster boards, cut into fourths and labeled as shown below.

Example Poster

Sticker Station A

1. _____	11. _____
2. _____	12. _____
3. _____	13. _____
4. _____	14. _____
5. _____	15. _____
6. _____	16. _____
7. _____	17. _____
8. _____	18. _____
9. _____	19. _____
10. _____	20. _____

Sticker Set Example

Sticker Station A

(1)	(2)	(3)
(4)	(5)	(6)
(7)	(8)	(9)

(10)   **USE EACH STICKER IN NUMERICAL ORDER**

Procedure:

1. Give each student in the class a set of ten numbered stickers of different colors, sizes, or shapes.

2. Strategically and quietly locate ten posters in different parts of your room (or throughout the school).

3. Tell the students to place their stickers, one at a time, and in order of one through ten, on any of the posters that they come across throughout the morning on the next available place on the poster.

4. Unobtrusively place one "germ" on one of the posters.

5. In the afternoon, collect the posters and display them in the front of the room.

6. Have the students who had placed a sticker on the poster with the germ, mark all their stickers that they placed on other posters.

7. Have the students who placed a sticker on one of the posters after a sticker of an "infected" person mark all their stickers.

8. Repeat for all stickers that apply.

9. Discuss the transfer of the "germ" and its implications.

10. Point to the need to wash off these germs.

(Step 10 could be extended by placing a "clean" sticker on a poster in the morning.)

ACTIVITY 3

Contagiousness

Educational objectives:

1. To illustrate the impact a sneeze can have on a room.

2. To further the understanding of germs and how they are transmitted from person to person.

Materials:

1. Balloons.

2. Different colored holes from paper hole punches.

3. Measuring tapes.

4. Graph paper.

Procedure:

1. Distrubute a balloon, a tape measure, graph paper, and a handful of paper punches to each group.

2. Have the students put the paper punches inside the balloon.

3. Instruct them to blow up the balloon.

4. In an open space, preferably on a tile floor, have the groups pop their balloons.

5. Instruct the students to find the paper punch that traveled the farthest, and measure the distance.

6. Repeat with the closest paper punch, and several other punches in all different directions.

7. Have the students graph their results.

Closure

Conduct a group discussion on the implications of the information collected.

ACTIVITY 4

Celebrate Our Differences

Educational objectives:

1. To allow the children to discuss and appreciate the differences among them, especially among people who have had the experience of living with an illness.

2. To enable the students to appreciate the needs of those with an illness and understand that their illness does not mean that they cannot enjoy the same things that other people enjoy, including friendship.

Materials:

- Chart paper.
- Markers.
- Materials to make silhouettes: lamp, black and white paper.
- Construction paper.

Procedure:

1. Have the students, in groups of four or five, draw a composite of what they believe a perfect student looks like. (Model this first for younger students.)

2. After the drawings are complete, have the groups choose one of their members to share their composite with the class. Have them explain how they developed their drawing and what makes their character "perfect." Display the drawings around the room.

3. Lead a discussion on whether anyone fits these composites. (Does anyone match the ideal? Are there any two people exactly alike? Do our differences make it harder or easier to get along with each other?)

4. Ask the students to list several people whom they admire. (Are these people alike?)

5. Introduce the idea that many of the world's heroes have had some kind of illness or disability. (Helen Keller–blind and deaf; Ludwig van Beethoven–deaf; Albert Einstein–learning disabled; Theodore Roosevelt–polio; Magic Johnson–HIV/AIDS; Jacquie Joyner Kersee–Asthma)

6. Discuss how these people overcame their individual challenges.

7. Make silhouettes of each other, or poems, to celebrate the differences in the class.

Silhouettes are created by using a lamp, which is shined on a wall. Allow the students to cast their shadows onto a piece of white paper hanging in the light. Have a partner trace their shadows. The students then cut out their shadows and paste them on a black piece of paper.

Acrostic poems of the students' names can be written. Have the students write their names vertically down the left side of a sheet of construction paper. Help them write and illustrate a poem, each line of which begins with one of the letters of their name. For example:

P—Perfectly silly

A—Always happy

M—Mostly adventurous

Closure

Have the students share their silhouettes and poems. Afterwards, reinforce the concept that we must celebrate our differences. Point out that everyone, not only students with an illness, is different, and that we must be careful to respect, value, and understand each other.

ACTIVITY 5

Warning Signs

Educational objectives:

1. To develop an understanding of the warning signs that the student with a illness may exhibit.

2. To practice how to react to these warning signs.

Materials:

The list of warning signs found in the appropriate chapter.

Suggested activities:

1. Have the students role play situations in which warning signs are exhibited and the proper reactions are given.

2. Present each warning sign. Brainstorm on the ways in which these signs manifest themselves, and how to appropriately help a classmate exhibiting these signs.

3. Have the students make a poster that depicts the different warning signs. (Younger students can cut and paste pictures from magazines.)

Extensions:

1. Spend some time discussing or reading about the idea of respect.

2. Practice emergency procedures. (911 emergency phone number, SOS emergency signal.)

3. Create a "game station" within the classroom that provides activities for students with restrictions.

4. Have the class brainstorm on what an emergency looks like, using role play, charades, or Pictionary.

Chapter 8

First Aid

Anyone who has spent time with children knows that there is no such thing as being too prepared. At school, there are minor injuries or situations that a teacher is expected to handle. School districts often have policies concerning the first aid care of students. Unfortunately, these policies are not always made available to classroom teachers. Clinic personnel or district nurse consultants can usually provide the necessary information upon request. Of course, any serious situations should require an immediate call to emergency services.

One of the easiest ways to increase safety within a classroom is to add a first aid kit to the class supplies. The kit should be separate from any daily classroom supplies, such as Band-Aids and tooth containers. The supplies in the kit must be current and readily available, in order to be effective in a emergency.

The following is a short list of the supplies that could be the basis for a first aid kit in the classroom. Each teacher should add to this list any materials specifically needed for the geographical area in which the school is located or those supplies potentially needed by the students with special needs. (snake or insect bite serum, emergency Allergy shot, glucose tablet, etc.).

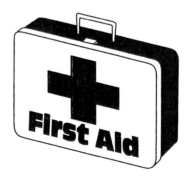

- cotton gauze bandage
- Band-Aids (assorted sizes)
- bandanna
- cotton balls
- bottle of water
- antibacterial ointment
- string
- needle and thread
- paper and pencil
- Vaseline
- scissors
- safety pins
- flashlight (with batteries)
- tape
- tourniquet
- cold pack (empty ice bag)
- blanket (for shock)
- sugar/glucose tablets/ can of juice or pop
- disposable latex gloves
- Poison Control Center phone number
- coins for a pay phone (in case of a field trip emergency)
- school phone numbers
- student emergency phone numbers
- sunscreen

Many districts do not allow the use of anything other than soap, water, and gauze bandages on wounds. Check with your district to see if calamine lotion and antibacterial ointment can be included in your kit. They are useful additions.

School field trips are an important consideration when putting together your first aid kit. It may determine the type of box or bag that you use to contain your supplies. Backpacks are a useful option. They are small, portable, and easy to grab in a hurry.

FIRST AID STEPS

The following are some basic steps to follow for minor first aid. It is important to remember that the safest, and smartest way to deal with a situation that is obviously not minor, is to call for assistance from emergency services.

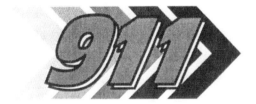

Call 911 if any of the following symptoms appear:
- severe difficulty swallowing;
- tight feeling in chest or throat;
- difficulty breathing;
- serious bleeding;
- unconsciousness;
- very high fever;
- very cold and clammy skin;
- or if you are unsure what is happening.

Bleeding

- Use a clean bandage or material to apply pressure to the wound.
- Clean the wound with soap and water.
- Raise wound above the heart, if possible.
- Apply firm pressure between the heart and wound.

Bruises (Including a black eye)

- Apply ice or ice packs.

Burns

- Apply cold water immediately (for at least 10 minutes).
- Do not apply butter or lotions!
- If burn is serious, call for help.

Choking

If the person is choking and unable to breath

- stand behind student;
- make a fist with one hand;
- reach around the student;
- place fist just below the student's ribcage;
- grab fist with other hand;
- with short, quick, upward strokes, apply pressure under the ribs.

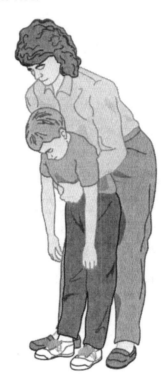

Cuts

- Apply pressure until the bleeding stops.
- Clean cut with soap and water.
- Cover with a clean bandage.
- If signs of an infection appear, notify the parents or doctor. (These signs include: pus, a spreading redness around the area, red streaks radiating from the cut, or swollen glands.)

Dizziness and/or Fainting

- Lay person down and raise their feet, or have them sit with their head between their legs.
- Apply a cold cloth to the forehead.

Frostbite

- Warm area quickly with warm water.

Head Injuries

- Call 911 if serious.
- Lay person down.
- Watch them carefully (for nausea, vomiting, dizziness, unequal pupils, slurred speech, inability to arouse).
- Record suspicious behavior for emergency services.
- All head injuries should be reported to the parents.

Heatstroke

- Try to lower body temperature (with cool water; cold, wet cloths; by fanning; etc.).

Insect Stings and Bites

- Carefully remove stinger, if present. (Do not use tweezers or fingernails.)
- Clean area with soap and water.
- Apply ice.

Nosebleed

- Sit person forward, so blood does not run down throat.
- Do not tilt head back.
- Pinch the end of the nose for 3 to 5 minutes (breath through mouth).
- If two different attempts are not successful in stopping the bleeding, call 911 or a physician.

Poisoning

- Call 911.
- If directed, cause the child to vomit.
- Collect some of the poisonous material to take to the hospital.

Seizures

- Push nearby objects out of the way.
- If possible, roll person onto their side (so saliva drains out—to prevent aspiration).
- Try to keep area safe.
- Loosen clothing around neck.
- Do not try to prevent their movements.
- Keep them on their side.
- Allow them to rest or sleep until they are alert (this may be several hours).
- Time the seizure—if it lasts more than a few minutes minutes or if multiple seizures occur—call 911.

Shock

- Symptoms: pale face; cold, sweaty skin; fast breathing; rapid and weak pulse; nausea, anxiety.
- Lay student down.
- Cover them with a blanket.
- Elevate legs.
- Call for help (911).

Sprain or Suspected Fracture

- Do not move person.
- Apply ice to area.
- Elevate injury, if possible.

Sunburn

- Apply cold pack.

⌁⌁⌁⌁⌁ Appendix A

STUDENT DATA FILE AIDS

To effectively care for a student with a serious illness, the school must be fully informed of that child's needs. In most cases, parents are prepared beforehand by medical professionals and approach the school administration with information in hand. If the information has not been presented to the school, however, it must be requested. A sample letter of request, along with a formal information card for the student, follows. An anecdotal record is also included. This can be used to keep track of the student's symptoms or side effects observed during the school day. It can also be used upon the request of the family or medical personnel to assist in the diagnosis.

REQUEST FOR INFORMATION

Dear Parents,

I am aware that your child _____ has _____.
I realize that this condition means that they have some special needs. To ensure that your child receives the proper attention while at school, please supply us with the necessary information by completing the enclosed information card. We are also requesting a copy of any record-keeping forms that may need to be filled out during school hours. If there is any additional information that you believe would be helpful for us during the school day, please add your comments to the information card.

Student Information

Name ――――――――――― Teacher ――――――― Grade ――

Condition ――――――――――――――――――――――

Parents ――――――――――― #'S ――――――――――

――――――――――― #'S ――――――――――

Doctor ――――――――――― #'S ――――――――――

Other ――――――――――― #'S ――――――――――

Medications

Name	Side Effects	Warning Signs	Dosage	Time

Snacks or Special Diet Needs ――――――――――――――

――――――――――――――――――――――――――

Tests ――――――――――――――――――――――――

――――――――――――――――――――――――――

Emergency Plan ―――――――――――――――――――

――――――――――――――――――――――――――

Anecdotal Record Keeping Sheet

Name of Student _____

Grade Level _____ Age _____

Date	Time	Notes

REQUEST FOR PERMISSION

The child's parents are responsible for providing the school with the necessary information concerning their child's illness. The teacher, however, can make a formal request for this information. The preceding materials will help teachers to make such a request. Asking the parents' permission for the other adults working with the child to be made aware of the child's illness and the health concerns involved is not mandatory. However, requesting parental permission to share with the class that a child is suffering a serious illness is necessary. The following is an example of such a request.

Dear Parents,

I would like to teach _____'s classmates about his illness. I plan to give an overview of the facts about _____ as well as teach lessons on the warning signs of which we should all be aware in the classroom for _____'s safety, the vocabulary associated with the illness, and some aspects of the human body that are involved. I will approach this as a unit of science. If you would allow me to share this information with the class, please sign below. If you have any questions about my plans, or any suggestions that may help in this endeavor, please call me at school.

Thank you,

I give my permission for the class to study _____.

Signed_____ Date_____

～／～／～／～ Appendix B

ORGANIZATIONAL CHECKLISTS

Items to Request from the Parents
- ☐ emergency information
- ☐ information on medicines and their side effects
- ☐ individual warning signs for their child

Materials Needed to Care for the Child During the School Day
- ☐ medicines
- ☐ test-taking supplies
- ☐ snacks
- ☐ official record-keeping material
- ☐ pillow, blanket, and cot for rest period (the school may supply these)

Locations for Student's Information
- ☐ classroom
- ☐ clinic
- ☐ office
- ☐ substitute's folder
- ☐ field trip folder

The People Who Need to Be Informed
- ☐ office staff
- ☐ specials teachers (P.E., art, music)
- ☐ media specialist
- ☐ recess aid
- ☐ cafeteria aid
- ☐ other adults who will be responsible for the child during any school day

What They Need to Know
- ☐ warning signs
- ☐ information locations
- ☐ side effects
- ☐ symptoms

⌐⌐⌐⌐ Glossary/Index

Note: numbers after entry indicate page numbers where further discussion may be found.

AIDS (Acquired Immune Deficiency Syndrome) 55–61, 64, 65, 73, 96
A severe disorder that eventually destroys the immune system. It is caused by the Human Immunodeficiency Virus (HIV).

AZT (zidovudidne and azidothymidine) 58
An antiviral drug used in the treatment of HIV/AIDS.

Acyclovir 58
A synthetic, or man-made, treatment for infections.

Agglutination 57
A clumped mass caused by like materials sticking to each other.

Albumin, 17
Proteins found in blood and other living tissues.

Allergen 1, 2, 4–6, 12, 13
The substance that causes a particular allergic reaction and stimulates the production of Antibodies.

Allergy 1-5, 7
An abnormal sensitivity to harmless substances.

Anaphylactic Shock 1, 2, 5, 13
A sudden, severe, and potentially fatal allergic reaction.

Anaphylaxis 1–3, 5
An acute allergic reaction that involves the entire body.

Anemia 73–75, 78, 83
A condition in which the body has an abnormally low number of red blood cells.

Angiography 30
An examination of the blood vessels used in the diagnosis of cancer.

Antibody
A protein produced in the blood that identifies dangers and alerts the body's defenses.

Antigen 57
A substance that, when introduced into the body, stimulates the production of antibodies.

Asthma 15–18, 20, 22, 24, 25
A chronic respiratory problem marked by breathing difficulties, chest tightening, and coughing.

Asymptomatic 57, 65
The state of having no symptoms of a disease.

Benign 27, 28, 31, 40
Of no danger, noncancerous.

Biopsy 30
The removal and examination of tissue that is suspected to be cancerous for the purpose of diagnosis.

Bone Marrow 27, 28, 30, 32, 37–40
A sponge-like tissue that fills most bone cavities and produces red blood cells, white blood cells, and platelets.

Bone Marrow Aspiration 30
A procedure in which a sample of bone marrow is removed through a needle in order to study it.

Bone Marrow Transplantation 32, 39
A procedure in which destroyed bone marrow is replaced by donated bone marrow.

Bronchi 15, 16
The two main branches of the trachea, or windpipe, leading directly to the lungs.

Bronchioles 15, 21
The tube-like extensions of the bronchi.

111

HIV (Human Immunodeficiency Virus) 2, 3, 55–61, 63–65, 73, 96
The retrovirus that causes the Acquired Immune Deficiency Syndrome.

Hemoglobin 74, 78
The oxygen-bearing, iron-containing protein in red blood cells.

Hemophilia 72, 73, 77, 82
A hereditary disorder characterized by excessive and sometimes spontaneous bleeding.

Hemorrhage 28
Severe, uncontrolled bleeding.

Hereditary 73, 77
Genetically transmitted.

Hormones 57
Chemicals produced by glands in the body that control the actions of certain cells or organs.

Immune System 1, 2, 9, 13, 32, 55, 65, 73, 75, 77
The complex group of cells and organs that defends the body against infections and diseases.

Immunosuppressed
The state in which the body's ability to fight infection is decreased. This occurs after chemotherapy and administration of large doses of radiation.

Immunotherapy 5, 12, 13
A method of treating cancer in which substances that stimulate the body's immune system are used.

Incubation 57
An infection's period of development, from the time of its entry into an organism up to the time of the appearance of the first symptoms.

Infection 1, 13, 16, 19, 28, 29, 32, 33, 40, 55–60, 65, 70, 73, 75, 102
The invasion of disease-producing organisms into the body.

Insulin 41–46, 48, 49, 53, 54
The hormone produced by the pancreas that enables cells to burn sugar.

Ketoacidosis 44, 54
A state in which not enough insulin is available in the body. Blood sugar is usually high at this time.

Leukemia 27–30, 32, 37, 38, 40
A disease in which bone marrow switches from making mature white blood cells to making a large number of immature white blood cells.

Leukocytes (WBC) 28, 40
White blood cells. The cells in the blood that aid the body in fighting infection and in developing immunity.

Lymph 27–30, 40, 55
The fluid that travels through the Lymphatic system, carrying cells that help fight infection and disease.

Lymphatic System 27
The tissues and organs, including the bone marrow, spleen, thymus, lymph vessels, and lymph nodes, that produce, transport, and store cells that fight infection and disease. This system has channels that carry lymph.

Lymph Nodes 28, 29, 55
Bean-shaped structures scattered along Lymphatic vessels. The nodes act as filters, collecting bacteria or cancer cells that may travel through the Lymphatic system.

Lymphocytes 55
White blood cells that produce substances to fight bacteria, fungus, and viruses.

Lymphoma 27, 28, 29, 40
Cancer of the Lymphatic system.

Magnetic Resonance Imaging (MRI) 31
A procedure involving a magnet linked to a computer that creates pictures of areas inside the body.

Malignant 27, 28, 40
Cancerous. Threatening to life or health.

Metastasis 27, 35, 36, 40
The spread of cancer from one part of the body to another.

Minor Motor Seizures 69
> A type of epileptic seizure.

Myeloma 27
> Cancer of the bone marrow.

Myoclonic Epilepsy 69
> An uncommon form of epilepsy seen in young children.

Partial Seizures 68, 69, 77
> A form of epilepsy.

Petit Mal Seizures 68
> Another name for Generalized Nonconvulsive Seizures.

Platelet 28, 30, 40
> One of the main components of the blood. They form clots to stop bleeding.

Pneumonia 16, 58, 59
> An acute or chronic disease marked by inflammation of the lungs, and caused by viruses, bacteria, and physical or chemical agents.

Psychomotor Seizures 68
> A type of epileptic seizure.

Radiation 31, 32, 39, 58
> The emission and multiplication of waves or particles of energy.

Radioactive 17, 31
> The state of exhibiting spontaneous emission of waves or particles of energy.

Radionuclide Scanning
> An exam that produces pictures of internal parts of the body. The patient is given an injection or swallows a small amount of radioactive material. A scanner then measures the radioactivity in certain organs.

Retrovirus 55, 62, 63, 65
> A virus that is capable of instructing a healthy cell to produce the virus along with itself when the cell reproduces.

Sarcoma 27
> Cancer of connective tissue, such as bone, cartilage, fat, muscle, nerve sheath, or blood vessel.

Seizure 67–70, 77, 79, 104
> A sudden convulsive attack.

Sickle-cell Anemia 73–75, 78, 83
> A hereditary condition characterized by the presence of oxygen-deficient sickle shaped cells, episodic pain, and leg ulcers.

Side Effects 33, 105, 106, 109
> Problems that occur when treatment affects healthy cells.

Stimuli 67, 77
> Something that causes a response.

Symptomatic 57, 65
> The state of showing indications of a disease.

T-cell Lymphocyte 55
> A white blood cell that functions in the defense against diseases.

Temporal Lobe Seizures
> A type of epileptic seizure.

Thrombocyte 28, 40
> A blood platelet.

Transfusion 56, 73, 78
> The direct injection of whole blood, plasma, or another soluble into the blood stream.

Tumor 27–31, 40
> A mass of excess tissue.

Ultrasound 31
> A diagnostic technique in which pictures are made by bouncing sound waves off organs and other internal structures. Tumors are identified from these pictures.

X-rays 17, 30, 31
> High-energy radiation used in large doses to treat cancer, or in low doses to diagnose the disease through pictures of the internal body.

‒‎‎‎‒‎‎Bibliography

Altman, Roberta, and Micheal J. Sarg, M.D. 1992. *The Cancer Dictionary: An A to Z Guide to Over 2,500 Terms.* New York: Facts on File.

Children's Hospital AIDS Program. n.d. *Caring for Your Child with HIV/AIDS.* New Jersey: Hoffman-La Roche.

‒‒‒‒‒‒. n.d. *HIV/AIDS: An Overview.* New Jersey: Hoffman-La Roche.

Du Bose, Estelle G., and Barbara L. Bowker. 1994. *The Life Process: Grief Recovery.* Littleton, CO: Life Process Publishing.

Epilepsy Foundation of America n.d. *Epilepsy: You and Your Child.* Landover, MD: Epilepsy Foundation of America.

Joseph, Lou, and John J. Lynch. 1990. *Allergy: Fact or Fiction.* Chicago: Budlong Press.

‒‒‒‒‒‒. 1990. *Diabetes.* Chicago: Budlong Press.

Kestler, Darryl, ed. 1993 *MacMillan Health Encyclopedia.* 6 vols. New York: MacMillan.

Moshé, Soloman L., M.D., ed. 1993. *The Parke-Davis Manual on Epilepsy.* New York: The KSF Group.

National Institutes of Health. 1993. *The Immune System, How It Works.* Bethesda, MD: National Cancer Institute.

‒‒‒‒‒‒. 1993. *Young People With Cancer: A Handbook for Parents.* Bethesda, MD: National Cancer Institute.

National Jewish Center. 1992. *Your Child and Asthma.* Denver CO: National Jewish Center for Immunology and Respiratory Medicine.

‒‒‒‒‒‒. 1989. *Understanding Allergy.* Denver CO: National Jewish Center for Immunology and Respiratory Medicine.

‒‒‒‒‒‒. 1989. *Understanding Asthma.* Denver CO: National Jewish Center for Immunology and Respiratory Medicine.

Netter, Frank H. 1989. *Atlas of the Human Body.* Summit, NJ: CIBA-GEIGY Corporation.

Zydlo, Stanley M., Jr. M.D., and James A. Hill, M.D. 1990. *The American Medical Association Handbook of First Aid and Medical Emergency Care.* New York: Random House.

About the Author

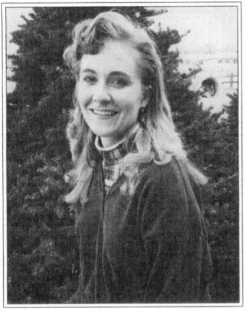

Andrea Mesec is a fourth grade teacher in Jefferson County, Colorado. She received her B.A. at Duke University in North Carolina and an M.A. in Curriculum and Instruction at the University of Colorado. Currently, Ms. Mesec is pursuing her dream of earning her private pilot's license. Andrea is a native of Colorado, who loves a good book, as well as winter, spring, summer, and fall in the Rockies.

Edwards Brothers Malloy
Thorofare, NJ USA
January 8, 2014